G000079520

Abortion Care as Moral Work

Critical Issues in Health and Medicine

Edited by Rima D. Apple, University of Wisconsin–Madison and Janet Golden, Rutgers University–Camden

Growing criticism of the U.S. healthcare system is coming from consumers, politicians, the media, activists, and healthcare professionals. Critical Issues in Health and Medicine is a collection of books that explores these contemporary dilemmas from a variety of perspectives, among them political, legal, historical, sociological, and comparative, and with attention to crucial dimensions such as race, gender, ethnicity, sexuality, and culture.

For a list of titles in the series, see the last page of the book.

Abortion Care as Moral Work

Ethical Considerations of Maternal and Fetal Bodies

Edited by Johanna Schoen

Rutgers University Press

New Brunswick, Camden, and Newark, New Jersey, and London

Library of Congress Cataloging-in-Publication Data

Names: Schoen, Johanna, editor.
Title: Abortion care as moral work: ethical considerations of maternal and fetal bodies /
   edited by Johanna Schoen.
Other titles: Critical issues in health and medicine
Description: New Brunswick: Rutgers University Press, [2022] | Series: Critical issues in
   health and medicine | Includes bibliographical references and index.
Identifiers: LCCN 2021039250 | ISBN 9780813597263 (paperback) | ISBN 9780813597270
   (hardback) | ISBN 9780813597287 (epub) | ISBN 9780813597294 (mobi) |
   ISBN 9780813597300 (pdf)
Subjects: MESH: Abortion, Induced—ethics.
Classification: LCC HQ767.15 | NLM HQ 767.15 | DDC 179.76—dc23
LC record available at https://lccn.loc.gov/2021039250

A British Cataloging-in-Publication record for this book is available from the British Library.

This collection copyright © 2022 by Rutgers, The State University of New Jersey

Individual chapters copyright © 2022 in the names of their authors

All rights reserved

No part of this book may be reproduced or utilized in any form or by any means, electronic
or mechanical, or by any information storage and retrieval system, without written permission from the publisher. Please contact Rutgers University Press, 106 Somerset Street, New
Brunswick, NJ 08901. The only exception to this prohibition is "fair use" as defined by U.S.
copyright law.

Sara Dubow's article originally appeared as "'A Constitutional Right Rendered Utterly
Meaningless': Religious Exemptions and Reproductive Politics, 1973–2014," *Journal of
Policy History*, Volume 27, Issue 1, January 2015, pp. 1–35. DOI: https://doi.org/10.1017
/S0898030614000347.

The article "Dangertalk" originally appeared as Lisa A. Martin, PhD, Jane A. Hassinger,
MSW, Michelle Debbink, MD, PhD, Lisa H. Harris, MD, PhD, "Dangertalk: Voices of Abortion
Providers," *Social Science & Medicine* 184 (2017):75e83.

References to internet websites (URLs) were accurate at the time of writing. Neither the
author nor Rutgers University Press is responsible for URLs that may have expired or
changed since the manuscript was prepared.

⊖ The paper used in this publication meets the requirements of the American National
Standard for Information Sciences—Permanence of Paper for Printed Library Materials,
ANSI Z39.48-1992.

www.rutgersuniversitypress.org

Manufactured in the United States of America

This book is dedicated to all of those who fight to preserve women's access to quality abortion care. And to Terry Beresford and Morris Turner who are missed.

Contents

Abortion Care as Moral Work

Introduction

Providing Abortion Care

Women of all backgrounds have experienced unwanted pregnancies, and many of them sought an abortion even when the procedure was illegal. In 1966, journalist Lawrence Lader investigated the consequences of illegal abortion. In the mid-1950s, estimates of the number of illegal abortions ranged anywhere from 200,000 to 1.2 million a year. Among urban White, educated women, one-fifth to one-fourth of all pregnancies ended in abortion, but only about 8,000 abortions annually took place inside a hospital, constituting a fraction of the number of abortions performed each year.[1] Women without resources, Lader noted, were forced to enter a world of underground abortions where care was frequently humiliating and the procedures dangerous. "Its practitioners, preying mainly on poor and ignorant women, rarely have a medical degree," Lader cautioned— many had occupations as clerks, barbers, and salesmen.[2] Before the mid-1960s, the estimated mortality rate from illegal abortion stood at 1,000 to 8,000 deaths per year. Almost 80 percent of all abortion deaths occurred among non-White women.[3] Women with resources could visit a skilled abortion provider or travel to foreign locations for abortions; those without were the most likely to die of a botched abortion.

On January 22, 1973, the U.S. Supreme Court legalized abortion with its *Roe v. Wade* and *Doe v. Bolton* decisions.[4] The decisions overturned nearly all state abortion regulations existing at the time and expanded the fundamental right of privacy to include abortion. With the legalization of abortion and the simultaneous introduction of vacuum aspiration machines to perform first trimester abortions, a previously clandestine and dangerous procedure became safe, quick, and inexpensive almost overnight. As Americans witnessed the emergence of a growing network of abortion clinics, abortions that had previously been invisible, performed behind the curtains of private physicians' offices or secretly by underground providers, became visible. The number of legal abortions climbed from 744,610 in 1973 to over a million in 1975, while the estimated number of illegal abortions declined.

These developments had a dramatic impact on abortion mortality. The mortality rate due to abortion had hovered between sixty and eighty deaths per 100,000 cases in the decades prior to legalization, but it sank to 1.3 by 1976–1977. Legal abortion before sixteen weeks' gestation, the authors of a study on morbidity and mortality of abortion concluded, had become safer than any other alternative available to the pregnant woman, including continued pregnancy and childbirth.[5]

Many physicians interested in providing abortions had cared for women suffering from the complications of illegal abortion and had seen their patients die. They recalled their despair as they tried to save women's lives before they bled to death or died of overwhelming infections. "We had a ward of patients who we admitted during the weekend," one physician remembers of his time as an obstetrics and gynecology (ob-gyn) intern and resident. "You'd go up there and it would smell. They'd have a tomato soup discharge. I remember one patient and as fast as we'd put the blood in, it would run and fill up your shoes."[6] In addition, many physicians had been frustrated with a system in which women with money and connections could obtain a safe abortion from their private physicians while women without such resources ended up in the emergency department with complications from illegal procedures. "The poor pulled the innards out or got soap shot up inside them," a St. Louis physician commented.[7] Now these physicians hoped to establish services that offered safe and affordable abortions to all women.

And many of the women who found their way into the emerging field of legal abortion in the early 1970s had themselves experienced an illegal abortion, participated in underground abortion services while abortion was illegal, referred others to those services, or had friends or relatives with such experiences. Inspired by the emerging women's movement and frustrated with traditional medical care, which they viewed as patriarchal and paternalistic, they looked to the field of abortion care as an opportunity to shape a more feminist future in medicine. Both groups came together in the early 1970s to establish a new system of abortion care. At times uneasy allies—male physicians found young feminist women challenging and demanding while young women found male physicians patronizing and dismissive of their concerns—they nevertheless negotiated over different aspects of abortion care and established a broad network of abortion clinics that influences abortion services to this very day.[8]

The very ease and speed with which patients gained access to abortions after legalization was tied to the invention of vacuum aspiration. Vacuum aspiration machines, imported in the late 1960s from England, shaped the emerging field of abortion care and meant that the procedure became a simple and safe outpatient procedure. In the course of the mid-1970s, a diverse group of physicians, feminists, and business people established freestanding abortion clinics to cater to women who could now access the legal procedure. The number of physicians performing legal abortions climbed by 76 percent, from 1,550 in 1973 to 2,734 in 1979.[9] It also led to the emergence of freestanding clinics. In 1973, of 1,550 providers who performed more than five abortions per year, 81 percent practiced in a hospital setting and 19 percent in a nonhospital setting. By 1979, of 2,734 abortion providers, 57 percent practiced in a hospital setting and 43 percent practiced in a nonhospital setting.[10]

The most widely used method of terminating second trimester abortions in the early 1970s was saline instillation in which the physician withdrew amniotic fluid and replaced it with a concentrated salt solution, leading to miscarriage within 24 to 36 hours. However, saline abortions could be performed only after the sixteenth week of pregnancy, when the uterine cavity contained enough amniotic fluid to allow for the procedure. In the 1970s, this left a window of four weeks during which women were usually unable to terminate unwanted pregnancies. By the end of the decade, however, abortion providers had begun to turn to dilation and evacuation (D&E), in which the fetus is removed, generally in parts, through the cervix and vagina.

Following the 1977 establishment of the National Abortion Federation (NAF), which provided abortion providers and clinic staff with a forum for support and information exchange, abortion providers turned their attention to the development and refinement of abortion procedures. Over the next decade they created a scientific discourse surrounding pregnancy termination procedures that included the comparison of different procedures and the development of support systems and counseling techniques for patients and clinic staff. NAF began to sponsor continuing education seminars to encourage abortion providers to switch from instillation procedures to D&E and to develop supportive services for abortion providers and staff involved in D&E procedures.

What kind of abortion services women were to receive and how they experienced legal abortion depended not only on the kind of abortion provider a woman visited but also on the philosophical orientation and organizational structures that shaped abortion services inside the clinic walls. The legalization of abortion and opening of abortion clinics had a profound impact on women seeking to control their reproduction, many of whom had had experiences with illegal abortion. Patients were grateful to have access to legal and safe abortion services, and their responses were overwhelmingly positive. The demand for services resulted in an explosive growth of clinics. By 1980, many clinics had grown from new offices with a small staff to large clinics that offered a wide variety of services and served an increasing number of patients.

But with the legalization of abortion, the country also saw the emergence of an antiabortion movement and almost immediate attempts to reverse the *Roe* decision. In April 1974, fifteen months after the legalization of abortion, Assistant District Attorney Newman Flanagan charged Boston ob-gyn resident Kenneth Edelin with manslaughter for performing a hysterotomy, a second trimester abortion procedure akin to a cesarean delivery. Critics held that the charges were racially motivated—Edelin was African American—and represented an attempt by the Boston Catholic community to undo the gains made under *Roe v. Wade*. Indeed, the Edelin case became the first test case surrounding legal abortion. The trial juxtaposed two very different narratives of abortion. The prosecution charged that Edelin's action had killed a live baby. Edelin's defense attorney contended that Edelin had performed a medical procedure that was sanctioned by good medical practice and the law.[11]

Seeking to establish the fetus as a person, antiabortion activists constructed narratives that described the fetal experience of abortion and fetal death. As the antiabortion movement emerged in the early 1970s, antiabortion activists also began to disseminate fetal images. Combined with the fetal narratives, the images took center stage in the unfolding debate, drawing attention away from the pregnant woman and transforming the fetus into a baby. By 1975, these modern views of the fetus contributed to a jury verdict where feelings about an image trumped scientific understanding: after the prosecution in the Edelin trial introduced images of the fetus, Edelin was found guilty, although the judge later overturned his conviction.

Antiabortion activists spent the late 1970s and 1980s creating increasingly gruesome abortion narratives. The narratives described the abortion procedure as a heinous process that caused agony for the woman and an agonizing death for the fetus. They positioned the fetus as a baby who was being killed and the pregnant woman as a murderer. They produced a body of propaganda that was disseminated via prolife newsletters and magazines and in educational materials distributed on picket lines and at crisis pregnancy centers. The materials tapped into a store of narratives stretching back to the pre-*Roe* era that depicted abortion providers as greedy and unscrupulous murderers and women who chose to have an abortion as irresponsible and mentally deranged. Fetal images became a mainstay on picket lines and at marches. Protestors regularly brought preserved fetuses to antiabortion protests to confront women with the fetal bodies. These materials proved crucial to the recruitment of antiabortion activists, many of whom joined the movement in the 1980s after viewing the images and movies produced in the 1970s. And they served as a rallying cry to a growing number of militant antiabortion protestors who hoped to garner publicity and to provoke public action that might further discredit abortion.

Even as antiabortion narratives of pregnancy terminations were depicting abortion procedures in increasingly violent terms, protestors were escalating their aggressive strategies to intimidate patients and clinic staff. The picket lines in front of abortion clinics had been relatively small in the 1970s, but during the following decade they gradually grew, reaching into the hundreds after the rise of a new antiabortion group focused on direct action tactics: Operation Rescue founded by Randall Terry in 1986. Unlike their largely peaceful predecessors, demonstrators of the 1980s aggressively approached clinic staff and patients; armed with posters, plastic fetuses, and specimens in jars, they frequently screamed at patients and family members. They fetishized the fetus and systematically escalated antiabortion tactics.

In the early 1980s, antiabortion activists in Chicago developed a protest activity they termed "sidewalk counseling." Initiated to present abortion patients with information that would make them change their minds before they entered the abortion clinic, the strategy won prominence with the publication of Joseph Scheidler's 1985 book *Closed: 99 Ways to Stop Abortion*. Scheidler was an antiabortion leader who emerged in Chicago in the early 1980s; he was the executive director of Friends for Life and the founder of the Pro-Life Action League, a national antiabortion group based in Chicago. In the very first chapter of his book, Scheidler described sidewalk counseling as

> the single most valuable activity that a pro-life person can engage in. . . . Counseling goes to the very heart of the abortion problem. The problem of abortion is the problem of killing babies. They are killed in abortion clinics or hospitals or doctor's offices and pro-lifers go there to intercede for the baby's life. The aim of the Pro Life Action League and other activists groups is to get more people out on the streets to stand between the killers and the victims.[12]

Such counseling was urgent—Schneider compared it to trying to physically stop someone who has rushed into your living room to kidnap your three-year-old child—and, he claimed, it was effective. In one thirty-day period, he insisted in his book, half a dozen sidewalk counselors at a few clinics had been able to stop ninety women from having abortions. While Schadler noted that the sidewalk counselor had to know something about human nature to understand why a woman might decide to have an abortion, he emphasized there was no one right way to engage in sidewalk counseling.[13]

By the middle of the 1980s, the line between sidewalk counseling and regular protest activities became impossible to draw. Encouraged to think of the "rescue" of a fetus as equivalent to the rescue of a baby or toddler, some sidewalk counselors did anything they could think of to discourage women from entering the clinic. They blocked clinic entrances, yelled at women seeking to enter clinics, and attempted to show women dead fetuses. "We feel that it's important to visualize and to educate and inform people," said Reverend Norman Stone, who regularly traveled with fetal remains to abortion clinics, at a 1985 demonstration in St. Louis. "So, sometimes it takes this kind of demonstration to make that point."[14] Antiabortion activists regularly intimidated women, trying to scare them away from the clinic. "They started yelling at people to get their attention. They said hateful, hurtful things to people," a Planned Parenthood staff member recalled.[15] One sidewalk counselor explained to a couple he had intercepted how God looked at abortion: "Women who reject his gift, his children, he makes them barren, because women have become sterile out of abortion. That's obvious, that happens all the time." He added, directed to the woman, "I just want to let you know that the consequences of your decision is [sic], before God you have now become a murderer."[16]

Protestors harassed patients, clinic staff, and abortion providers. They blocked entrances in an attempt to dissuade patients and employees from entering clinics, and they followed them into the building. They wrote down patients' license plate numbers to contact them later, followed the patients home, or just showed up at the patients' homes. Antiabortion activists terrorized the abortion providers day and night. They threatened staff, waited for abortion providers at airports, followed providers in their cars as they traveled to and from work, and showed up at the homes of clinic administrators and abortion providers. Protestors built human barriers to block access to clinics and to prevent abortion providers from leaving their homes. They physically accosted administrators and abortion providers. Employees and abortion providers regularly received hate mail and harassing phone calls at both their clinics and their private residencies. Protestors leafleted abortion providers' home communities with "Wanted for Murder" posters and terrorized the providers themselves by sending daily letters describing how they would be tortured and killed.[17]

Along with sidewalk counseling, antiabortion activists also turned to the establishment of crisis pregnancy centers (CPCs) to educate women about the dangers of abortion and discourage them from terminating a pregnancy. Established to provide pregnancy options counseling in the early 1970s, these centers significantly increased in number in the early 1980s when antiabortion activists intensified their efforts to reach out to women seeking abortions. One estimate notes that at the end of 1984 there were at least 2,100 CPCs around the country, many of them established by conservative Christian foundations. They attracted potential patients with the promise of free walk-in pregnancy tests. During a thirty-minute wait for the test results, a staff member would show the woman a film or narrated slide presentation detailing the horrors of legal abortion. The CPC staff members drew on antiabortion narratives of women who now regretted their abortions and told stories of fetal death to convey the alleged dangers of abortion and scare clients away from abortion clinics. Narratives of agonizing pain and death—for the fetus and the pregnant woman—were a central part of this information.

CPCs sought to confuse women who were looking for an abortion clinic, and they were most likely to attract young women who found themselves pregnant for the first time. Most of these young women were determined not to let their parents find out that they were pregnant, and many of them sought an abortion alone or with the help of a boyfriend or girlfriend. Scared and intimidated by what lay ahead, they were an easy target for CPCs. They frequently did not realize that they had gone to the wrong place, failed to recognize that the counseling at CPCs was biased, and were too shy to just leave the fake clinic if they recognized their mistake. If patients were still determined to end their pregnancies after these scare tactics, the CPC staff tried to mislead and delay them by sending them to appointments with various prolife counselors and physicians.[18] Indeed, delaying the procedure until women could no longer obtain a first trimester abortion was a common tactic at CPCs. Staff at CPCs also called women who had been to their clinic at their homes and sent clergy to their homes in hopes of changing their minds. Not only did experiences with CPCs leave these patients extremely disturbed, their emotional condition after visiting a CPC increased their risk of abortion complications.[19]

On March 10, 1993, antiabortion activist Michael F. Griffin shot and killed abortion provider David Gunn outside Pensacola Women's Medical Services in Pensacola, Florida. The news of Gunn's death shocked the abortion provider community. The killing of David Gunn led to an immediate escalation of personally targeted harassment and violence against abortion providers. That year, antiabortion violence spiked with two murders or attempted murders, thirteen bombings, arsons, or attempted arsons, and 415 incidences of clinic invasions, assaults, vandalism, death threats, burglaries, and stalking.[20] The following year, antiabortion protestor Paul Hill murdered Dr. John Britton and his bodyguard James Barrett, and John Salvi killed two receptionists at Planned Parenthood clinics in Brookline, Massachusetts. Seven others were wounded in the 1994 attacks.[21] Since then, at least eleven people have been killed, including four doctors, two clinic employees, a security guard, a police officer, a clinic escort, and two civilians.

By the 1990s, the escalation of antiabortion protests and the protestors' increasing use of violence had significantly stigmatized and isolated providers and clinic staff. The number of physicians willing to provide abortions had declined significantly. From a high in 1982, when the country counted 2,908 abortion providers, the number fell to 2,582 in 1988 and to 2,434 by 1991— a 16 percent decline in less than a decade. In the 1990s, the decline was even more drastic: 1,819 providers remained by 2000, a 37 percent decline from 1982.[22] With the decline in providers, it also became more difficult for patients to access abortion services. This was further aggravated by legislators' attempts to increase the barriers to women's access to abortion.

Indeed, the Roe v. Wade decision also signified the beginning rather than the end of a protracted legislative and legal battle over access to abortion. As the antiabortion movement gained strength, activists set out to eliminate funding for abortion services, overturn the Roe v. Wade decision, and restrict women's access to the procedure. In 1976, antiabortion legislators in the U.S. House and Senate passed the Hyde Amendment, which restricted federal funding for abortion. As early as 1974, Missouri and Ohio legislators tried to impose a range of restrictions on abortion, including parental consent requirements for minors, a husband's consent to his wife's abortion, a ban on second trimester saline abortions, a twenty-four-hour waiting period, and hospitalization requirements for second trimester abortions. While in 1976, the Supreme Court struck down the Missouri and Ohio restrictions, by the late 1980s, the U.S. Supreme Court shifted away from its refusal to allow state-imposed restrictions to abortion and embraced a new vision in which states could now express an interest in fetal life. In the 1989 Webster v. Reproductive Health Services decision, the Supreme Court allowed states to second-guess physicians by imposing specific directions and restrictions on abortion services.[23] The shift away from physician authority to a stronger role of state legislatures in the performance of abortion was further strengthened in a 1992 decision, Planned Parenthood of Southeastern Pennsylvania v. Casey.[24] States wishing to impose abortion restrictions now simply had to demonstrate that the burden imposed on women's access to abortion was not "undue"—that is, placed no "substantial obstacle in the path of a woman seeking an abortion of a nonviable fetus."[25] In *Casey*, the justices permitted abortion barriers that the Supreme Court had found unconstitutional in previous cases: a twenty-four-hour waiting period, state-mandated counseling, parental consent for minors, and a reporting requirement. The court also began to treat women as a group who needed to be protected from their own choices. Over the following years, Supreme Court justices further expanded the restrictions on abortion. Most significantly, the 2007 *Gonzales v. Carhart* decision upheld the first ban on a particular abortion procedure—intact D&E or the so-called partial birth abortion procedure—without granting an exception to women's health or life.[26]

More broadly, for the past two decades states have drafted increasingly inventive legislation to impose all kinds of restrictions on abortion services, ranging from requiring particular building codes to the requirement that abortion providers have privileges at local hospitals to attempts to ban abortions after six weeks' gestation. None of these restrictions have increased the safety of abortion procedures, which were already the safest outpatient procedures available.[27] All of them made abortion services more difficult to access by placing obstacles in the way for women seeking abortion services or by forcing abortion providers to raise their prices to meet burdensome and costly requirements.

The contributions in this anthology will explore the historical context and present-day challenges to the delivery of abortion care. The contributing authors address the motivations that lead abortion providers to offer abortion care, discuss the ways in which antiabortion regulations have made it increasingly difficult to offer feminist-inspired services, and ponder the status of the fetus and the ethical frameworks supporting abortion care and fetal research. Together these essays provide a feminist moral foundation to reassert that abortion care is moral work.

Notes

1. Lawrence Lader, *Abortion* (Boston: Beacon Press, 1966), 17, 59.
2. Lader, *Abortion*, 64.
3. Lader, *Abortion*, 2–3, 66. Other estimates of mortality rates were even higher. One study at the University of California's School of Public Health estimated 5,000 to 10,000 abortion deaths annually. Almost half of all childbearing deaths in New York City were attributed to abortion alone. See also Cynthia Gorney, *Articles of Faith: A Frontline History of the Abortion Wars* (New York: Simon and Schuster, 1998), 23, 529, and Mary Streichen Calderone, ed., *Abortion in the United States: A Conference Sponsored by the Planned Parenthood Federation of America, Inc. at Arden House and the New York Academy of Medicine* (New York: Harper and Brothers, 1958). For an assessment on the links between state interference and safety of the

procedure, see Leslie J. Reagan, *When Abortion Was a Crime: Women, Medicine, and Law in the United States, 1867–1973* (Berkeley: University of California Press, 1997).

4. Roe v. Wade, 410 U.S. 113 (1973); Doe v. Bolton, 410 U.S. 179 (1973).

5. Willard Cates Jr. and David A. Grimes, "Morbidity and Mortality of Abortion in the United States," in *Abortion and Sterilization: Medical and Social Aspects*, ed. Jane E. Hodgson, 225–275 (New York: Grune and Stratton, 1981), 170.

6. Takey Crist, interview with Johanna Schoen, May 20, 2001, Jacksonville, NC. Such experiences powerfully shaped physicians' approaches to abortion once the procedure became legal. See, for instance, Carol Joffe, *Doctors of Conscience: The Struggle to Provide Abortion before and after Roe v. Wade* (Boston: Beacon Press, 1995), 53–69, and Gorney, *Articles of Faith*, 16–17, 217–218.

7. Cited in Gorney, *Articles of Faith*, 218. After legalization, this physician joined the medical staff of Reproductive Health Services, the first abortion clinic in St. Louis.

8. Carol E. Joffe, Tracy Weitz, and C. L. Stacey, "Uneasy Allies: Pro-Choice Physicians, Women's Health Activists, and the Struggle for Abortion Rights," *Sociology of Health and Illness* 26, no. 6 (2004): 775–796.

9. Alan Guttmacher Institute, Table 10, "Number of Abortion Providers by Provider Type by State, 1973–82, 1984–85, and 1987–88" (in author's possession).

10. Alan Guttmacher Institute, Table 5, "Number of Providers, Abortions, and Abortions per Provider by Type of Provider and Metropolitan Status, 1977–82, 1984–85, and 1987–88" (in author's possession).

11. As quoted in Kenneth C. Edelin, *Broken Justice: A True Story of Race, Sex, and Revenge in a Boston Courtroom* (Sarasota, FL: Pondview Press, 2007), 315.

12. Joseph M. Scheidler, *Closed: 99 Ways to Stop Abortion* (Rockford, IL: Tan Books, 1985), 19.

13. Scheidler, *Closed*. See also "Pro-Life 'Abortion Clinics,'" *Harper's Magazine*, December 1985, 25.

14. *Holy Terror*, directed and written by Victoria Schultz (Hudson River Productions, 1986), accessed in the Susan Hill Papers, Duke University Libraries Archives and Manuscripts.

15. As quoted in Alesha Doan, *Opposition and Intimidation: The Abortion Wars and Strategies of Political Harassment* (Ann Arbor: University of Michigan Press, 2007), 123.

16. Schultz, *Holy Terror*.

17. See Johanna Schoen, *Abortion after Roe* (Chapel Hill: University of North Carolina Press, 2015), chapters 5 and 6. For a firsthand account, see Susan Wicklund and Alex Kesselheim, *This Common Secret: My Journey as an Abortion Doctor* (New York: Public Affairs, 2007).

18. See Schoen, *Abortion after Roe*, 180–186.

19. Schoen, *Abortion after Roe*, 184–185.

20. Patricia Baird-Windle and Eleanor J. Bader, *Targets of Hatred: Anti-Abortion Terrorism* (New York: Palgrave, 2001), 351.

21. Baird-Windle and Bader, *Targets of Hatred*.

22. Stanley K. Henshaw, "Factors Hindering Access to Abortion Services," *Family Planning Perspectives* 27, no. 2 (1995): 54–59, 87; Stanley K. Henshaw, "Abortion Incidence and Services in the United States, 1995–1996," *Family Planning Perspectives* 30, no. 6 (1998): 263–270, 287; Lawrence B. Finer and Stanley K. Henshaw, "Abortion Incidence and Services in the United States in 2000," *Perspectives on Sexual and Reproductive Health* 35, no. 1 (2003): 6–15.

23. Webster v. Reproductive Health Services, 492 U.S. 490 (1989).
24. Planned Parenthood of Southeastern Pennsylvania v. Casey, 505 U.S. 833 (1992).
25. Melody Rose, *Safe, Legal, and Unavailable? Abortion Politics in the United States* (Washington, DC: CQ Press, 2007), 57–85; Carole Joffe and David Cohen, *Obstacle Course: The Everyday Struggle to Get an Abortion in America* (Berkeley: University of California Press, 2020).
26. Gonzales v. Carhart, 550 U.S. 124 (2007).
27. Reva B. Siegel, "The Right's Reasons: Constitutional Conflict and the Spread of Woman-Protective Antiabortion Argument," *Duke Law Journal* 57 (2008): 1641–1692; Cates and Grimes, "Morbidity and Mortality," 170.

Part 1

Providers

The essays in the first section tell of the factors that led medical professionals to become involved in the provision of abortion care and of their experiences providing services in an increasingly politicized field. Experiences with illegal abortion motivated both Dr. Marc Heller and Dr. Morris Turner to begin to offer abortion care while Terry Beresford, who spent much of her career training abortion counselors, entered the field of abortion care by chance. For a whole generation of physicians who entered medical school and internships in the postwar era, the experience of abortion was tied to memories of caring for women with abortion complications. Those memories were frequently frightening, involving treating women dying of blood loss or infection.

They also scoffed at a system which, by the 1950s, allowed women with financial resources access to abortions, but left poor women in the hands of illegal abortion providers. In the 1950s hospitals began to set up abortion committees to review women's requests for abortions and decide whether they were warranted. This highly structured process successfully regulated and limited women's access to abortion. As medical indications declined in importance, physicians increasingly turned to psychiatric indications to justify the termination of pregnancy. If a pregnant woman could successfully argue that her unwanted pregnancy made her want to kill herself, a psychiatrist's confirmation could make the difference between a negative and a positive decision of a hospital abortion committee. However, the system of psychiatric consultation and referral was clearly limited in its ability to assist women in gaining access to abortion. Seeking the help of a psychiatrist was expensive and time consuming. Psychiatrists also were quickly overwhelmed with patients seeking consultations for therapeutic abortions; at times such consultations became a charade, which frustrated both the psychiatrists and the women who went to see them.[1]

A number of factors converged by the 1960s to set the stage for abortion reform. Responding to medical complaints about the lack of clear legal guidelines, the American Law Institute, made up of attorneys, judges, and law professors, proposed a model abortion law in 1959 that would clarify the legal exception for therapeutic abortion and enshrine it in law along more liberal lines. During the following decade, legal and medical organizations promoted the law institute's model in state legislatures and in the media. Women's growing need for access to safe abortion services had become painfully evident to the medical professionals who were staffing the nation's emergency rooms and taking care of women who had obtained illegal abortions. Fears about the dangers of thalidomide and then the German measles (rubella) epidemic also played a crucial role in emerging reform efforts. By the end of the 1960s, feminists began to organize to put pressure on the medical profession and on state legislatures to repeal abortion laws.[2]

By the mid-1960s, state legislators across the country were debating abortion reform based on the American Law Institute's model law; in 1967 Colorado, North Carolina, and California became the first states in the nation to pass reform legislation, closely followed by Alaska, Hawaii, and New York.[3] In addition, two court decisions in the fall of 1969, *People v Belous* and *United States v. Vuitch*, led to abortion reform in California and Washington, DC.[4] Following the Washington, DC, decision, Dr. Milan Vuitch established an outpatient abortion clinic a few blocks from the White House; with the help of the National Abortion Rights Action League, he opened an outpatient clinic in 1971 called Preterm, which served as a model for the establishment of freestanding abortion clinics and as a training ground for physicians across the country.[5]

Although the introduction of vacuum aspiration machines made the establishment of first trimester abortion services relatively seamless, the situation was more complicated for women whose pregnancies were further along. The most widely used method of terminating second trimester abortions in the early 1970s was saline instillation, in which the physician withdrew amniotic fluid and replaced it with a concentrated salt solution, leading to miscarriage within twenty-four to thirty-six hours. However, saline procedures came with a host of problems. First, there was a four-week period in which women were too far along for a first trimester vacuum aspiration but not far enough along for the saline procedure. Then there were the risks and unpleasant side effects for the pregnant woman. Finally, the procedure could lead to the delivery of a fetus still showing signs of life. Such outcomes were rare—only 1 percent of abortions in the 1970s took place after twenty weeks of gestation, and only one in 4,000 of those resulted in a live birth. When live births did occur, most of the fetuses were so immature that they died within 24 hours. Nevertheless, such events were disturbing.[6]

Because physicians frequently left after performing the amniocentesis (the withdrawal of amniotic fluid) and inserting the medication to begin labor, nurses usually had to deal with the fetus. As the authors of a study on the emotional demands of midtrimester abortion procedures commented, "amnio abortions [saline instillations] are viewed by the nurses as the most upsetting experience which occur [sic] and a symbol of abandonment by the medical staff. The ward nurses' comments speak clearly to the point of being left to cope with an upset patient who delivers late at night. The nurses found the physical contact with the fetus particularly difficult."[7] Dr. Morris Turner and Dr. Marc Heller both speak about nurses who refused to participate in saline abortions or abortion care in general. The refusal of health care professionals to care for abortion patients traces back to the 1973 Church Amendment. Passed in the wake of *Roe v. Wade* and signed into law by President Richard Nixon as an amendment to the Health Programs Extension Act, the Church Amendment allowed individual physicians and federally funded institutions to refuse to perform abortions or sterilizations for reasons of religious belief or moral conviction.[8]

By the mid-1970s, some abortion providers began to look for alternatives to saline abortions—in particular, the use of laminaria, seaweed sticks that, if inserted into the cervix, will absorb moisture and dilate the cervix. Most physicians used manual dilation to dilate the cervix, inserting progressively larger metal rods (dilators) that widened the cervical opening until the physician was able to insert the suction cannula or curette to perform the abortion. Dilation by laminaria required that patients come to the clinic twice—once for the insertion of the laminaria and then the next day for the abortion procedure. But proponents of this method felt that it was less traumatic and led to fewer complications, thus outweighing the disadvantages.

The use of laminaria allowed abortion providers to slowly extend the gestational age past the traditional twelve-week cutoff. Their ability to meet unexpected challenges when performing abortions contributed to their confidence and skills and increased the willingness of some physicians to perform abortions at more advanced gestational ages. In the end, the refusal of an increasing number of nurses to assist in instillation abortions and the continued threat of lawsuits in cases where aborted fetuses still showed signs of life forced hospitals to either limit second trimester abortions or adopt the dilation and evacuation (D&E) procedure. By 1980, D&E had emerged as the most frequently used method of second trimester abortion.[9]

In March 1975, abortion providers and their supporters met in Knoxville, Tennessee, for the first national symposium on abortion since the *Roe v. Wade* decision. Over three days the attendees visited workshops on clinic administration and funding, legal responsibilities, pregnancy termination techniques, abortion counseling, and birth control. Following the meeting, a group of twenty-five participants from clinics across the country discussed the establishment of a national organization of abortion providers. They formed a committee to plan the creation of the National Association of Abortion Facilities (NAAF) which, committee members hoped, would function as a forum to exchange information, support research, establish standards for abortion clinics, and lobby on behalf of abortion providers.[10]

In May 1975, two months after the conference in Knoxville, NAAF founding members met in Cleveland to hash out the creation of a national professional organization. Differences over organizational goals surfaced as soon as members sat down. While independent for-profit providers sought to create a provider service organization, many of the nonprofit clinics and policy organizations, such as Planned Parenthood and National Abortion Rights Action League [NARAL], were primarily concerned with standards of care and abortion access. By the end of the meeting, a group of providers had split off and formed the National Abortion Council (NAC).[11] In November 1976, when NAAF held its first annual meeting, a small group tried to broker an agreement between the two organizations and in early 1977, after months of negotiations, the two organizations formed the National Abortion Federation [NAF]. When NAF held its first meeting in Denver later that year, members of seventy-five different clinics and organizations participated. Terry Beresford recalls the heady days and difficult negotiations of the formation of and early days at NAF. The organization brought together a wide assortment of individuals: members of feminist collectives, owners of for-profit clinics, and abortion providers from diverse backgrounds were joined by researchers, academics, lawyers, and policymakers. All gathered to negotiate the goals and direction of the new organization.[12] For many attendees these meetings were eye-opening and invigorating. They also contributed greatly to the education of members as they found their individual identities in this diverse group of people.

Since its formation, NAF has been the most important professional organization for many abortion providers and those who work in the field of abortion care. It has set and upheld standards, provided continuing education to its members, helped with security concerns, offered a place to connect with researchers and lawyers, and provided a space where health care professionals, marginalized and frequently stigmatized at other professional meetings, could talk openly about their work.

Dr. Morris Turner and Dr. Marc Heller both speak of the social disapproval they experienced as a result of working as abortion providers. With the increasing stigmatization of abortion, all health care professionals working in abortion care, but in particular abortion providers, were frequently ostracized by their health care professionals at their institutions and experienced harassment in their public and private lives. Particularly intimidating was the intrusion of antiabortion protestors into the private lives of abortion providers, as they protested in front of physicians' private homes and harassed the children of abortion providers. Worries about the safety of family members, then, always accompanied fears about abortion providers' own safety. But, as the essay by Dr. Marc Heller illustrates, the intimate details that led women to seek abortions served as a constant reminder of the importance of providing abortion care.

Race shaped the experience of abortion patients, providers, and clinic staff. Abortion providers and their patients noted the specific use of race-based arguments in antiabortion propaganda. Dr. Morris Turner explains that white protestors picked up black nationalist charges that abortion was a form of racial genocide when approaching African American patients and staff. But African American patients and abortion providers were unconvinced by the appropriation of race suicide arguments by white demonstrators, finding them incoherent and peripheral.[13] And both African American patients and providers drew on a civil rights tradition when they decided to face down crowds of screaming protestors.

To curb the escalating harassment of abortion providers, patients, and clinic staff, clinic owners across the country sought the help of the police and courts. In some cities, close collaboration with city officials and community support led to a productive relationship between clinic owners and the police. Claire Keyes, who ran the Alleghany Reproductive Health Center in Pittsburgh, for example, was careful to maintain cordial relations with members of the city council and the police chief. In turn, the local police precinct responded quickly when called and regularly assigned an officer to stand guard on procedure days.[14] Terry Beresford, who spent most of her life training abortion counselors and for a time served as director of Preterm, talks about her work and the positive experiences she had with the police in Washington, D.C., where she directed the Preterm Clinic.[15] But while some abortion clinics praised their local law enforcement officials, others were unable to get any help from the police. Up to a third of police officers ignored antiabortion activists who violated the law, and some even sided with the protestors. They offered antiabortion protestors coffee and told them to "keep up the good work."[16] On balance, police officers were more likely to do nothing than actively aid antiabortion protestors. In the majority of cases where law enforcement officials were uncooperative, officers failed to show up when called, failed to act on or lost complaints that clinics had filed, refused to search for explosive devices when called to a bomb threat, refused to enforce injunctions and merely watched antiabortion activities from the sidelines, even when protestors violated the law. At other times, officers enforced the law so slowly that antiabortion activists still achieved their goals, arresting protestors who closed a clinic to prevent its opening, for instance, but acting so haltingly that the clinic was closed for the entire day.[17] Police departments frequently excused their lack of action by claiming that they had to stay neutral.[18] The law, it was clear, was only as good as those who enforced it.

The shooting of David Gunn, the first abortion provider to be killed in 1993, deeply shook abortion providers across the country. Dr. Morris Turner reflects on the impact that the increasing violence had on him and his colleagues as they renewed their commitment to do this work.

Notes

1. Leslie J. Reagan, *When Abortion Was a Crime: Women, Medicine, and the Law in the United States, 1867–1973* (Berkeley: University of California Press, 1997); Johanna Schoen, *Choice and Coercion: Birth Control, Sterilization, and Abortion in Public Health and Welfare* (Chapel Hill: University of North Carolina Press, 2005), chapter 3; Carole Joffe, *Doctors of Conscience: The Struggle to Provide Abortion before and after Roe v. Wade* (Boston: Beacon Press, 1995); Johanna Schoen, *Abortion after Roe* (Chapel Hill: University of North Carolina Press, 2015), chapter 1.

2. Reagan, *When Abortion Was a Crime*, 216–245; Leslie J. Reagan, *Dangerous Pregnancies: Mothers, Disabilities, and Abortion in Modern America* (Berkeley: University of California Press, 2010); Lawrence Lader, *Abortion* (Boston: Beacon Press, 1966), 148.

3. Melody Rose, *Safe, Legal, and Unavailable? Abortion Politics in the United States* (Washington, DC: CQ Press, 2007), 6–7. See also David J. Garrow, *Liberty and Sexuality: The Right to Privacy and the Making of Roe v. Wade* (New York: Macmillan, 1994).

4. People v. Belous, 71 Cal.2d 954; United States v. Vuitch, 402 U.S. 62 (1971).

5. Lawrence Lader, *Abortion II: Making the Revolution* (Boston: Beacon Press, 1973), 115–120; Schoen, *Abortion after Roe*, chapter 1.

6. George Stroh and Alan R. Hinman, "Reported Live Births Following Induced Abortion: Two and One-Half Years' Experience in Upstate New York," *American Journal of Obstetrics and Gynecology* 16, no. 1 (1976): 83–90, https://doi.org/10.1016/0002-9378(76)90469-5, 83, 87; Schoen, *Abortion after Roe*, chapter 2.

7. Nancy B. Kaltreider, Sadja Goldsmith, and Alan J. Margolis, "The Impact of Midtrimester Abortion Techniques on Patients and Staff," *American Journal of Obstetrics and Gynecology* 135, no. 2 (1979): 235–238, https://doi.org/10.1016/0002-9378(79)90351-x, 237.

8. Public Law 93–94, 93rd Congress, 1136. See also Lisa H. Harris, "Recognizing Conscience in Abortion Provision," *New England Journal of Medicine* 376, no. 11 (2012): 981–983, https://doi.org/10.1056/nejmp1206253.

9. In 1981, 9.7 percent of all abortions were performed after the first trimester, 64 percent were performed by D&E. By 1988, that number had climbed to 87 percent with 10.5 percent of abortions taking place after the first trimester.

10. Terry Beresford, interview with Johanna Schoen, September 30, 2012, Alexandria, VA; "A History of the National Abortion Federation," n.d., file NAF History, Terry Beresford Papers, Sally Bingham Center for Women's History and Culture, Duke University Libraries, Durham, NC.

11. "History of the National Abortion Federation."

12. For more on the founding and role of the National Abortion Federation, see Schoen, *Abortion after Roe*, chapter 3.

13. Schoen, *Abortion after Roe*, 176; Morris Turner, interview with Johanna Schoen, October 6, 2013, Pittsburgh, PA.

14. Turner, interview with Schoen, October 6, 2013.

15. Beresford, interview with Schoen, September 30, 2012.

16. Rochelle Sharpe, "Clinics Get Little Support from Officials," *Abortion: The New Militancy*, Gannett News Service Special Report series, December 1985, 11, file NWHO, General Reports, Rochelle Sharp, Police Response, Susan Hill Papers, Duke University Libraries Archives and Manuscripts.

17. Sharpe, "Clinics Get Little Support," 11.

18. Sharpe, "Clinics Get Little Support," 12.

Chapter 1

A Narrative

Morris Turner

I grew up in South Georgia. My parents were sharecroppers. I can remember as young as I was, I had this yearning to be a physician. This was at a time of intense segregation. At the doctor's office, there was the Colored waiting room and the White waiting room. And the Colored patients were seen after the White ones. My mother was intensely ill and in lots of pain, but she had to wait until the White patients had been seen. And as a young kid I remember thinking: If I were a doctor I would do it differently. I can remember writing a term paper in ninth grade about how I wanted to be a doctor and about my philosophy.

I was delivered at home. My aunt delivered me. This was a rural area. Midwives delivered at home; the doctor came by some time later. These were not trained midwives. They would come by and do whatever they could. I remember several young women dying from complications of pregnancy. Getting pregnant out of wedlock was a no-no. You were thrown out of church; you were thrown out of school; the word spread. And that impressed me. I remember one of the senior high school students walking across the stage and a week later delivering a term baby. She had hid the pregnancy all the time because she wanted to finish school. But back in those days you were thrown out.

I went to Morehouse College in Atlanta. During the time my wife and I were dating—this is 1966, 1967—there was a young woman who was pregnant, and the pregnancy was unwanted. She had gone some place for an illegal abortion, and she died at Grady Hospital of overwhelming sepsis. And I remember, back in the day, when some young family member had gotten pregnant, they would buy quinine over the counter. They knew if you took enough of this, you could sometimes cause an abortion.

I went on to medical school at the University of Pittsburgh. This was 1971 or 1972. I was doing rotations through obstetrics and gynecology. And at that time, abortion was in the news. There was an incident here in western Pennsylvania at West Penn Hospital. I knew that they were doing some abortions in the hospital; but you had to have two physicians, one of which had to be a psychiatrist, to attest to the necessity of the abortion. There was a district attorney, Bob Duggan, who was strictly antiabortion. A young woman who was on the brink of dying underwent an abortion beyond the first trimester—it may have been late in second trimester. Doctor Leonard Laufe performed this abortion. This was before *Roe v. Wade*, and a nurse reported this to the district attorney's office, who then brought charges against Dr. Laufe. That made headlines at least here in western Pennsylvania. But Dr. Laufe was never found guilty.

As a medical student, you had to do rotations through the emergency room. There were a number of patients who presented to the emergency room from various places who had undergone illegal abortions. To this day, I am not sure what people did. You hear about the coat hangers. They'd come in bleeding with puncture wounds in their cervix, and they'd be infected. And we had to take care of them. The patients wouldn't tell you where they came from.

I remember one young lady totally bleeding. At this time I was a senior student on a rotation through the emergency room. And she came in pregnant and just bleeding, bleeding, bleeding. And my resident with whom I was working went in to see her. She had lots of blood and lots of pain. But when we cleared all of the blood out of the vagina, there were several little pieces of what looked like charcoal in her vagina. Neither of us had seen this or knew what it was. But our staff physician, Professor Margulies, who later became chairman of the department at McGee,[1] came down and immediately recognized that this was something called potassium permanganate that somebody had put in or had given it to her to put in. And this stuff had eroded her vagina—whatever place it touched, it went through. So the bleeding was not coming from the pregnancy, it was coming from her vagina; the pregnancy was still intact. We had to take her to the operating room to flush out all those pieces and sew her up to stop all that bleeding. And then she certainly qualified, from a psychological standpoint, for a therapeutic abortion. That was probably the most dramatic one that I remember seeing before *Roe v. Wade* and before the start of Women's Health Services.

In July 1973, I started my residency. My interest naturally drew me to abortions. There were residents more senior to me in the program who would do the abortions on those patients who had gone through the abortion committee and had been declared in medical need of an abortion. As a resident in the hospital, I learned to do the vacuum aspiration procedure under general anesthesia.

The biggest abortion case was in Boston: Kenneth Edelin in 1974. The Edelin case left a big impression, not only on me but also on the department and chairman because we were doing abortion procedures. The outcome was going to affect any program that was doing abortions. But it was even more impressive to me that Edelin was an African American at Harvard, that he was the chief resident. That made much more of an impression on me than that he was being charged with manslaughter for performing a saline procedure. Wow, he's gotta have all kinds of credentials. We followed that case very, very closely.

Women's Health Services was the first outpatient abortion clinic in Pittsburgh, set up by Tom Allen and Leah Sales. Tom knew how to do vacuum aspirations. They held the clinic three days a week: Tuesday, Thursday, and Saturday. At the time they only did first trimester, as an outpatient, up to twelve plus weeks, less than thirteen weeks. And they did over a hundred patients a day when it opened in 1973. We had three or four physicians working, all at the same time. Leah, a social worker, set up the counseling. It was a big operation. We had the lab and then the procedures and the recovery. Even though now I am a resident, it was a totally different process performing abortions at an ambulatory site. That's pretty much where we all learned how to do them. Those of us interested in doing procedures under local anesthetic had to moonlight. They put you through a training process, and then eventually you worked there.

I also learned to do saline procedures during my residency. We never did them prior to *Roe v. Wade*. When I began my residency, those residents who were interested could rotate on that service where we provided saline abortions. That was the only way to provide second trimester abortions; we had a unit in the hospital dedicated to salines, and there were lots of salines. There were nurses at the hospital who didn't want to be part of that—they didn't want to participate. In fact, there were only two, maybe three nurses of all the staff who would serve on that unit. And then at some point [1982], *Casey* brought about a state law that said you can't force nurses to do that.[2] They can object and don't have to lose their job. The hospital had to look specifically for nurses who would do saline abortions.

At Women's Health Services, initially it was just the first twelve weeks. And then gradually, with experience, we began to do more and more. And then finally we went up to fourteen weeks. That lasted a while until we gained a lot of experience with that. I learned to do dilations and evacuations (D&Es) in the hospital from the senior residents who had been taught by someone before them and they just passed it down. But then I learned to do it as an outpatient procedure with Allegheny Reproductive Health Center. That was 1974. I was pretty much self-taught—just gradually moving up until you had a number of them under your belt and you became proficient. As we learned how to do the D&E as outpatient, there were still some saline abortions. I can remember doing them up until the late 1980s, early 1990s.

We were able to develop our services and make them safer and safer. Initially, we didn't use laminaria. Laminaria wasn't part of the scene until late in the process. First was the development of the dilators—the metal dilators. And then came the concern for damage to the cervix and how you can prevent that. That's when the idea of laminaria developed and later on more advanced things like Lamisil and Dilapin.[3] But first was the laminaria. With the creation of the National Abortion Federation (NAF), word spread on how you can do these.

When Dr. Richard Suite became chairman of the department, he came from San Francisco where they had been doing the late second trimester D&E, and he brought Mitch Crenin with him. And as chairman of the department, he pretty much laid down the law of the land: that this is what we would do. It was so much more efficient to do it that way. With salines, you had to bring patients in, and you had to instill them; they stayed overnight, and you had to have nursing personnel to stay with them. It was much more costly to do that as opposed to D&E. He pretty much laid that out. Now that we had people who could do them proficiently, it shifted it from the floors, where you had to have a unit for the saline procedures, now to the operating room. The same principle applied: you had to have those willing to assist with procedure even in the operating room. But that seemed to find much more favor; you had many more people involved with that than with saline. Then you pretty much had a regular crew that you knew and could rely on to be there. So in many ways that eased the process.

In the early 1970s no one had raised the issue of Black genocide. Most of the patients were White. Almost all of the women we saw in the emergency room were Black. The editor of the *Pittsburgh Courier* was one of the most prominent persons to declare that abortion was Black genocide. That raised the question in the community. I couldn't ignore it. But at that time I didn't have to respond because I was performing abortions at an institution; and so it was more of an institutional thing, and I was covered. When I finished my residency in 1976, however, my partner and I started performing abortions in an office—same procedure, except that you could do it on private patients. Patients didn't have to march through demonstrators. Now it's not an institution anymore; it's my practice. The community knows that I am providing abortions. And I think the saving grace was that it was provided safely, discreetly, and it was a private matter. There were a number of people who took advantage of this. Whether they were pro or anti or whatever, no one had to know about it. I found the secrecy a little bit disturbing, but nevertheless, I was committed to patient safety and patient privacy. So whatever their thoughts were, patients came to get this done. Many White patients as well.

And then, in 1982, the Pennsylvania Abortion Control Act required that you had to register with the state health department as an abortion provider. *Casey* involved getting spousal and parental consent. Nobody could come from out of state—some really horrendous imposition on women at that time. And a lot of the White physicians pulled away from that because they had a lot of their business in obstetrics, delivery of babies. And many of their patients would not come to them if they knew they were doing abortions. So they started referring them either to agencies or to us because they didn't want to face the problems from their private patients. In the Black community there were one or two people who charged Black genocide, yet the patients kept coming and defending the fact that "this is a private matter between the doctor and myself" and that "this is none of your business."

Claire Keyes introduced me to NAF around 1980. I found comfort in the organization. I could go and there were people on the stage talking openly about how to do abortions. That was unheard of. You could go to the American Congress of Obstetricians and Gynecologists, and you could go to other things, and you might hear a roundtable discussion, and you'd only have four or five people. Here was an open conference with a room full of people who had the same ideas and the same end result about providing safe and legal abortions across the nation. It was very reassuring, and you gained knowledge. Initially there were people from the Centers for Disease Control. They coordinated to bring out the statistics. They would put out these reports [on the] status of abortion in America. David Grimes was one of the ones in charge. One of the first NAF conferences I went to was held in Atlanta. I've been to a number—I went to one in Pensacola shortly after David Gunn was killed. People were nervous about that. And then I also went to one in St. Louis, which was a real big one. And then there was one here in Pittsburgh and New York.

I first became aware of protest activities at McGee, before I started working in the outpatient clinics. They were marching around McGee with their signs: Stop Abortion Now! They would march around the hospital. However, I didn't have any contact with them until I started working at the freestanding clinics— now you actually gotta pass through them in order to get to work. My office was in the Medical Center East. And Allegheny Reproductive was on Highland

Avenue, right where it crosses Penn Avenue. And that's about three blocks from where my office was, where I would park and then you had to walk there. And so anywhere along the route they'd take pictures of you. They knew who we were. They often had your picture on their signs. And they used that as propaganda all over. "This is the abortion provider"—on the sign. They knew all of us. And they ultimately found out our home addresses and our office addresses. So there were occasions when they would demonstrate outside the office. They've been on the street here [at the Morris family home], and certainly in front of the clinic, every session, every session.

Initially, it was a little unnerving because they were yelling at you: "Murderer! How could you do this? These women are suffering!" I always had trouble figuring out what they meant. Women freely come to get these procedures done based on what their perceived needs were. But somehow we were making them suffer. And that was always their theme: stop these women's suffering. They'd yell all kinds of names at you. Then they'd have some of the more radical . . . usually some men that were involved in the process, who would actually come face to face with you to impede your way. Again, a little bit unnerving. But the more you did it, the more you got used to it, and the more you expected it. And then, of course, along the way there were physical fights. Some of the men who were accompanying their women to the procedure—protestors would approach them, and sometimes tempers flared, and you would actually have physical confrontations.

I never engaged because the one thing that I learned early on is that you couldn't talk to them reasonably. There were physicians on the staff at McGee who vehemently opposed doing abortions. There was a group there that was very Catholic in their convictions, and they just didn't want anyone to do it. Of course, they would always try and get the hospital not to allow abortions to be done, but they were never successful. But there were occasions when we would try to meet with them to discuss the issue. What is it that you don't see? These women are coming to get this; they tried to get it even when it wasn't legal. So what is the problem? And we learned early on that there was no reasonable exchange. They were convinced in their belief that this should not occur under any circumstances, that it is taking a life. And therefore there is no reason, even in the gravest of illnesses, that you ought to do this.

Channel 2 here, the CBS affiliate, had a program or two—talk shows—where they had both sides on stage. And even they learned that when you presented facts and you tried to talk practical things, it just went totally past them. You could not get exchanges with them. The answer was always the same. So we learned early on, the providers, there is no talking to them. Then they started setting up these bogus phone lines, advertisements: come see us if you want alternatives to pregnancy, talk about adoption, we'll do an ultrasound. People didn't realize until they went that this was an antiabortion proposition. They just wanted to get them in and tell them how sinful it was. They had big signs all over: "Alternative to abortion." It also became evident that sometimes these people can go off their rocker. You saw doctors being killed.

The killing of Dr. Gunn was totally unexpected. They used the bible and religion as their backbone, so you figured they wouldn't do anything like that. But then you saw those things to interrupt the process [i.e., pictures of protestors locking themselves to cars], and that's when you realized the Gunn incident was essentially the culmination of all the things. They can literally go off their rocker. That's when Dr. Kisner decided, "I am not going down without taking somebody with me." Those were his exact words. He got a gun. But I didn't. I was never a gun person.

The murder of Dr. Gunn scared the hell out of me, especially when you wake up one Saturday morning and the whole street out here is full of demonstrators. They went to Dr. Kisner's house at Fox Chapel. On one occasion they actually came up to the lawn. That's when we had to get the police involved. Their idea was to arouse the neighbors and let them know I live here. To my pleasant surprise, the neighbors took up arms to get them out of here. That sort of shocked them. Most of my neighbors were Jewish. Particularly in the Jewish community it is well known that they had had abortion providers for years before this discussion about legal versus illegal. So when these demonstrators came down in here, it was no big deal to my neighbors that I lived here because I was a servant as far as they were concerned. And don't you dare come down in here—that was an affront to my neighbors, and that certainly helped take care of that situation. There was this law that you could not demonstrate if there were no sidewalks, and if you are going to be on the street, you need to go down and get permission from the city. This was when Mayor [Sophie] Masloff was in administration. But the other places [the home neighborhoods of physicians where antiabortion activists would demonstrate] had sidewalks, so unfortunately protestors could do it there.

I was extremely worried [about my kids in school]. My kids went to school at St. Bede's school, two blocks down. They walked to school. That bothered me. I loved the school. There were no nuns there; they were all lay teachers. There were certainly Catholic leaning teachers, but there was the priest who was the head of the diocese who knew me, knew what I did. For some reason, he never harassed my kids. We worried about that. These were my boys, and they were not going to take being harassed. My oldest son was in fourth or fifth grade when he went to St. Bede's. They were small, but they were never approached.

On one occasion, there was a parent–teacher conference at the school. And the priest, who was head of the school, made it a point when he was on stage presenting to talk about abortion. This is a parent–teacher conference—it has nothing to do with abortion or with the function of the school and what the kids were doing. I was in the audience, down in front. You know, we are not in a church, and 60 percent of the students enrolled here are not even Catholic—and that was keeping the school open. But that's what he chose to do; and in the middle of his presentation, I got up and walked out, making noise as I was leaving. There were several other parents who followed me, and we all gathered outside.

I was surprised that he had the audacity. It never happened again. Ultimately, someone caught him somewhere, in a park. He had someone [i.e., was having an affair with a woman]—obviously it wasn't a wife—and he had two kids.

The principal got on well with my kids. All of my kids were very athletic and participated in the athletic program there. They were valued. All the parents knew us. They knew us for obvious reasons—because we were the only Black family there. I got along very well with that whole group, the elementary school.

Now comes high school: Central Catholic High School! By this time, the Catholic church had the names and pictures of all of us providers. They knew who we were. So here, my oldest son going to Central Catholic, welcomed with open arms. There was this Brother David—who knew who I was, knew what I did—but [for him] this is about kids. I really admired him for that because he was true to his conviction. All people are god's creation. The kids were not doing this, this was on me. My oldest son said, on one occasion—maybe his sophomore, junior year—there was one teacher in the school who brought up my name to him on one occasion, aside, not in a public area. But it never happened again. And then four years later my twins came through. They never had any run-in with anybody there.

And the most ironic thing: there was this set Catholic rivalry with another school on the north side—North Catholic and Central Catholic—the Catholic World Series, if you will. Once a year they played, and all of the Catholics in Pittsburgh came. They were playing in North Park. One of the referees on the field had a heart attack while the game was going on, and I was in the stand. I am not a cardiologist; I am an ob-gyn. The staunch Catholics—and there were doctors that I knew sitting in the audience—never made one move to go out and see about the guy who was laying in the field. And one of the administrators at the school looked up and saw me and kind of beckoned if I would come. And so, of course, I went out and started CPR [cardiopulmonary resuscitation] on him, and I rescued him. Before I got there, though, there was a priest there who was giving him the last rites—they had written him off. And here comes this Black abortionist out of the stand of all these Catholic hosts—and their kids all sitting around. And there was I, on the field, saving this guy. I rescued him. The ambulance came, and they took him.

My kids never had one word said to them. They knew my kids. But all was forgiven—many of their wives and daughters came at some point to get an abortion. Their restrictions were meant for other people.

The people who protested were always the same. You knew them. I could spot someone who was not a regular. And those are the people that I always watched when I was on my way. The regulars I could judge. I knew what they would say; they had been there forever and ever. These newer ones—you never knew whether they were recruited in or whether they were just using the regular demonstrators to gain access to us. And that was always a worry because you just couldn't look around every corner. The security guards, we certainly knew them up close and personal. And they would often meet us. There was a time when we received threatening mail, at which point we would report it to the FBI, and they would come and interview us and talk to us; for a while they'd come around on provider days, clinic days. But obviously they couldn't sit there the whole time.

Claire [Keyes] was very instrumental in staying in the politics of it. She knew the city council representative for our district. She would know the commander of our local police station and could talk to them and would befriend them. And so they would assign someone for three or four hours just to sit on clinic days, to make sure that nothing out of the ordinary happened. That made us feel better. There was an occasion where I came to my office on a Saturday— to the office building, the fourth floor—you take the elevator up. When I got off the elevator, the hallway was filled with these demonstrators, just blocking the door. I couldn't get to my office. The police had to come and escort them. They were chained to each other, handcuffed; my office staff had already called the police. They were all arrested, packed in the paddy wagons, and taken downtown.

That then caused us to have to hire a security guard for the office because there were occasions where they would come up and have a seat in the waiting area, like they were a patient. And then another would come in, talking to the "patient." They would try all kinds of things. Then you had to get a security guard to sit in front of the office in order to prevent that. That was a little bit intimidating to some patients, too: Why do you need a security guard? Patients were loyal, though. And for the most part, they realized that we were performing a function requested of us. And over the years, eventually they [i.e., the protestors] were locked up and given fines, and that tactic kind of went to the wayside. The leaders—Randall Terry and several other people—ended up going to jail, and not just for a little while. They were there for about a year. And so, because they didn't have leaders—people who had previously sacrificed, had gone to jail, and they had been fined and had criminal records—fewer and fewer wanted to volunteer. That helped to ease the situation, but it also brought out the crazies; the ones who stayed were more apt to do something harmful. That made it very, very touchy at that point.

The counselors who would first have contact with patients who had been demonstrators, who had stood on the picket line, they let them know: "We've seen you on the line out there. And for our purposes, we need to know why you are here. And how do you reconcile how you go from the line to now wanting to have this done?" That happened not infrequently. Sometimes you think they'd do that just to get access, and [they'd wait] right up to the moment of the procedure and then change their minds; and that gives them information, and they can go back. But that never happened; [instead] they went through with the abortion procedures with the thought "I need this. Unlike the others, I really, really need this." But by this time we had realized that their sense of reasoning is not what you and I would accept as reasonable. [But] we never turned them away. I can't recall ever refusing anybody.

You can count the Black protestors on one hand. Over all the years there was one lady, who still occasionally comes. I never took the time to talk to her, but she was coming from a religious standpoint, [and she] reads bible verses. And the thing that really seems to frustrate them is that I don't acknowledge their presence. It's as if they don't exist. And they just can't stand that. They shout things at you. But I don't engage them. I did look at her at one occasion, as if to say, "Why are you here? Have you seen any other Black people out here?" Although it was never a verbal communication. There were no Black churches in Pittsburgh that were strongly antiabortion. The Black church with the largest congregation is Mt. Ararat [Baptist Church], whose ministers have all known. My wife is a deacon at that church. And a number of people at that church referred [patients] to us through their counseling process. There have been a number of churches throughout the city whose pastors have openly referred patients to us. I thought that was telltale: here were practical people, and then we can deal with whatever convictions they had, or guilt, afterward. But this is what patients need. And the ministers would openly defend what we were doing. I thought that was fantastic. We would have a list of the ministers around the city who were open minded about the process and who often served as counselors post abortion. We could refer patients back. They have youth congregations where I go to present slides on sexually transmitted diseases, and I've been welcomed in those instances. They realize that people need access.

All my life, I've been privileged to provide services for people. I've just become so resolute in this that I figured if those people are out to get you, it'll happen. They have so much opportunity to do that. And if I walked around every step of the way worrying about it, then I would be totally disabled. I never bothered going to get a gun; it just precipitates more violence. I've become resolute—not complacent, but resolute. If it's meant to be, that's what will happen. I always take in the landscape, every time I walk across that street, to see who is there, what is there, to see if I can see what is coming. But if it is coming, there is really not much I can do to stop it.

But then, here is a doctor, George Tiller in Kansas, who is in church, ironically with a bulletproof vest on.[4] There is no protection you can take against that. And yet there was no satisfactory resolution to that whole process. That is just such a violation of human rights. There is no defending against fanatics. That was as sad a story in American history as it can get. That's as sad as lynching. It's home grown. That is a sad, sad commentary. A man in church, having to wear a bulletproof vest to protect against ideology.

Notes

1. University of Pittsburgh Medical School's Magee-Womens Hospital.
2. Planned Parenthood v. Casey, 505 U.S. 833.
3. Lamisil and Dilapan are synthetic dilators.
4. George Tiller worked as an abortion provider in Wichita, Kansas, where he ran Women's Health Care Services. He gained national prominence as one of a handful of physicians to provide abortions late in pregnancy. Many of his patients sought his help because they were carrying fetuses with fetal abnormalities. On May 31, 2009, Dr. Tiller was shot and killed by antiabortion extremist Scott Roeder while Dr. Tiller served as an usher during Sunday morning service at his church in Wichita. Roeder was convicted of murder on January 29, 2010, and sentenced to life imprisonment.

Chapter 2

Being an Abortionist

Marc Heller

I am an abortionist, and being an abortionist is about stories. Being an abortionist means that every time I leave for work, my wife gives me a hug, and says, "Drive safely." It's our code for "Be careful."

Being an abortionist means always wondering how to respond in social situations, when someone asks, "So, what do you do?" Lately, I've started to have the courage to say, "I'm a gynecologist, but mostly I do abortions." If I'm lucky, they reply, "I'm pro-choice, but I don't believe in using abortion as a method of birth control. Those women should be more responsible." "And the men?" I might reply. *Silence.* But once I've "confessed," they often say, "Do you do 'late term' abortions?" I tell them I go to about four months. "Why do they wait so long?" they ask, with a slight sneer. I tell them that it's mostly because there are no longer many places to get an abortion. *Silence.*

Being an abortionist means ignoring the protestors outside my clinic every day: the seven-foot-high statue of the Virgin Mary, the sign with the huge disarticulated fetus. They scream at the staff: "You have blood on your hands." "You are f-cking whores." They scream at the patients: "We'll take your baby!" "Don't kill your baby!" A recent caller to the clinic said, "You f-cking murderers! You baby killers! Your doctor deserves to die." So I always enter at the rear door of the clinic, be sure I have my entry fob in my hand before I get out of my car, and walk quickly to the steel reinforced door.

Being an abortionist means that I know my patients have just been terrorized by our protestors. I greet each one before they get undressed. I shake their hand, I look them in the eye, and I smile. I say, "We'll take good care of you today." I always say "we" because, just before she inserts the intravenous line, the sedation nurse says, "Hi! I'm Donna. I'll be your bartender today." And during the procedure, after they're usually somewhat sedated, Christina says, "You have such beautiful eyelashes," or "Is your hair naturally wavy? It's beautiful. I'd die for hair like that!" or "You better start thinking about where you want your boyfriend to take you to eat. You'll be out of here in forty minutes. Is he a good guy? Do you have someone to pamper you today?"

Being an abortionist means helping a woman who came with bruises all over her arms and face, and a Band-Aid on her pinkie because her boyfriend just pulled out her fingernail with pliers. She was eighteen weeks pregnant. "I can't believe it," she said. "He was never like this before." "Are you safe?" I asked. "Yes, I'm moving to my mom's house in Florida." Afterward, she asked, "Can I see it?" "Of course," I replied, "but it will be in pieces." I showed her the fetus. "Can I hold it?" she asked. I handed it to her, and she cupped it in her hands. "Oh, look at its little hands and feet. It had a penis . . . it was a little boy." She stared at it and said, "I'm sorry. I'm so sorry." She handed it back to me, and said to me, "Thank you *so much*. I love you."

Although I always warn them about what they are going to see, which of course depends on gestational age, I have no ambivalence about showing my patients their fetuses. This is primarily because of a terrible mistake I made when I was an intern in 1973. I had just delivered the baby of a sixteen-year-old. Her baby had a meningomyelocele, with part of its brain hanging out of the back of its head. It was squeaking. Its face was deformed, and its eyes were bulging. Just looking at it terrified me. My patient asked if she could see her baby, and I said no. The nurse whisked it away, and out of the room. I saw her again ten years later. She said to me, "Doctor Heller, you did the worst thing anyone has ever done to me in my life. You didn't let me see my baby." My patient died of AIDS two years later.

Being an abortionist means performing an abortion on a pregnant sixteen-year-old with a nine-month-old at home, whose boyfriend was in prison for robbery. She lived with eleven people in a three-bedroom apartment. When one of the nurses commented that it didn't seem she'd have much privacy, she said, "We make it work." And I immediately recalled one of my first deliveries when I was only an intern with three days' experience, one of the thousands I performed over the subsequent years. She was also sixteen years old. I heard her screaming from my on-call room, even before the page. "Doctor Heller to the labor room, stat!" "Take this f-cking thing out of me—take it out, you f-cking b-tch!" she said to the nurse. "Who the f-ck are you?" she said to me as I rushed into the labor room—and just managed to catch a wriggling, healthy, screaming boy. The baby was fine in spite of my inept efforts! Relieved, I called out to her and to the whole room, "It's a boy!" She looked away in disgust, "Oh no! A boy? Wait till I tell Billy!" Billy was drunk at a local bar. He never came to see her. We used to keep patients four days back then. She watched cartoons as she bottle-fed her baby. She never made eye contact with her child. Her baby was admitted three months later because he had gained only two pounds. "Failure to thrive," they called it. It took the nurses two days to get the crusted feces off the sores on his tiny bottom.

Being an abortionist means that I recall other parents who were going to keep their baby. That's always supposed to be OK. "God's gift," they call it. At one prenatal visit, the father pushed his eight-year-old son down the hallway. He said, "Come on, you shit, you worthless piece of shit." He wore one of two baseball caps to his wife's prenatal visits. One said "BOHICA—Bend Over, Here I Come Again." His wife's name was Dawn, so the other hat said "I'm so horny, even the crack of dawn looks good." In those days, family members usually waited outside when the chaperone and I did a pelvic exam. He always refused to leave. As I inserted the speculum, I could feel his hot breath on my neck. "Nice c-nt, huh?" he said.

Being an abortionist means helping a thirty-five-year-old woman who had three children and was happily married for fifteen years. Her ten-year-old middle child had recently died of intestinal obstruction that was misdiagnosed as the flu. After three months, her husband said, "I want to replace our son." She told me, "He didn't help me at all, and I told him that I'm not ready!" They had used the rhythm method [of birth control] successfully for years; her husband forced her to have sex during her fertile time. She said, "I'm so angry! I'm so angry! I have four children, and now I've lost two of them! My husband doesn't know I'm here. I'm going to tell him I had a miscarriage."

Being an abortionist means helping a college student who had great sex with a really hot guy she met in a bar. She'd had a little too much to drink. He didn't look so great the next morning. "I feel so dirty," she said. "So what did you do?" I said. "You had sex!" We see this, right? People don't think of other things when they're having sex, especially if it's good sex. What's the saying? "No one wrote the Great American Novel during orgasm!"

Being an abortionist means helping another college student with a great boyfriend. She wanted to go to law school before having kids. "I feel so irre-sponsible," she said. I always think, "Remember the penis!" But I usually say, "As I recall, it takes two to get pregnant."

Being an abortionist means performing an urgent abortion on a twenty-year-old with a two-year-old at home. Her leukemia had been in remission since she was fourteen, but she just relapsed, and they need to start chemotherapy immediately. I spoke with her hematologist on a Tuesday. He said, "By Friday, I will have wiped out her bone marrow with chemotherapy. Her chance of another remission is very slim. I doubt she'll make it."

When I decided to become an abortionist, I left the institution where I had practiced for thirty years—my professional home. One reason was because of an event that happened when I was there. I was helping a twenty-four-year-old, whose father had just died of malignant melanoma. She had a two-and-a-half-year-old at home, and brain metastases from *her* melanoma. Just before the case, the anesthetist walked by and said loudly, "I'm not doing it: I don't believe in them." My patient's neighbor, who she hardly knew, had brought her because she had no one else to help. She staggered as we helped her onto the stretcher and said, "I'm really sorry, but I can't walk very well. It's the tumors in my brain." It was the day that President [George W.] Bush first signed the so-called Partial-Birth Abortion Act of 2003.[1] I remember that picture of him sitting at his desk in the Oval Office with a bunch of smiling old men standing on either side of him. At first, we thought my patient might be fifteen weeks pregnant, which would have meant that she was in the second trimester of pregnancy. No one knew what the act would mean, so no second trimester abortions were being performed anywhere in New York state. The chief anesthetist was a fundamentalist Christian, and there was a fundamentalist Christian orthopedic surgeon who used to prowl the halls. In any case, only a few operating room staff would help me with abortions. Luckily, an ultrasound that morning confirmed that my patient was only nine weeks along; so I didn't have to face the dilemma about whether I dared to proceed.

At that same hospital, I ordered a preoperative sedative for a terrified sixteen-year-old, but the nurse didn't give it. The anesthesiologist had to put her to sleep on the stretcher before we could move her to the operating table because she was terrified—writhing, crying, gasping for breath. When I asked the nurse why she hadn't given the pre-op medication, she replied, "I was busy . . . and besides, I have no sympathy for women who get themselves in this position."

At that same hospital, I performed a late abortion on a patient with a fetus who had Down's syndrome. In those days, the results of genetic testing were only available later in pregnancy. She told me, "I just couldn't take care of this baby. I have a lot of trouble with depression. Life's already too hard for me." Post-op, she had a rare life-threatening complication. She asked me over and over, "Doctor Heller, am I going to die? Please don't let me die." She recovered completely after four days in intensive care. At her postoperative checkup, she told me that she had asked one of the nurses, "Is God punishing me?" "Yes," the nurse had replied.

Being an abortionist means that, after fifteen years, I received a referral for an abortion from a Christian fundamentalist ob-gyn colleague. During the intervening years, he had sent me a number of referrals for patients who needed help because they were carrying dead babies in their uterus, late in pregnancy. This patient had a seizure disorder, which had been well controlled for a year on multiple medications, but she started having seizures again as soon as she became pregnant. She was carrying twins. After I performed the abortion, he sent me the following text: "It took me some time initially to understand, but I have grown to know and appreciate how important what you do for women really is. I thank you."

Most of all, being an abortionist means always remembering my own mistakes, weaknesses, and imperfections, including my history of alcoholism and recovery. In 1986, I performed a technically difficult hysterectomy. I was hung over, irritable, and impatient. My patient's operation took six hours instead of three because I cut her ureter. I repaired it, and she went home in three days without any long-term problems. It's still hard for me to talk about: November 5, 1986, the day I had my last drink. When a sober alcoholic comes for an abortion and looks worried when she tells us about her history of addiction but has solid sobriety (I can always tell—it takes one to know one), I sometimes talk with her about myself. I say, "I'll judge you when I live a perfect life. I'm in recovery, too—twenty-nine years." I usually end with, "Hey, at least you know your doctor's sober!"

Being an abortionist means remembering the bus driver who drove me down an alley fifty-four years ago when I was twelve and made me jerk him off. So when a patient clamps her legs together as I try to put her in stirrups, I say, "Why don't you sit up so we can talk? Have you ever been raped or abused?" If she says yes, I'll sometimes tell her a bit about my own story. I say, "I'll treat you with the greatest respect. I haven't just read about this in books." I thought of my bus driver when I took care of a fifteen-year-old patient who was raped repeatedly by her twelve-year-old mentally challenged brother. She had very irregular periods, so it wasn't until the second trimester of her pregnancy that she realized she was pregnant. "I can't even brush my teeth," she told me. "He breaks my toothbrush."

And I always think of my bus driver when our local Catholic bishop leads his yearly protest march of the faithful past our clinic. I wonder how many twelve-year-old altar boys he's f-cked.

When I care for a patient with a history of panic attacks and anxiety and depression, I think of my lifelong struggle with depression. I often say, "Panic attacks are terrible, aren't they? I used to have them when I was in med school. You're afraid you're going to live, and afraid you're going to die! I'll be extra careful with you . . . We'll get through this together. No surprises. OK?"

Being an abortionist means remembering my wife's legal abortion in 1972. It had just become legal in New York State. We were still dating. We had no clue, but her IUD [intrauterine device] had slipped down into her cervix. After the procedure, her doctor said to me, "She bled a lot, but they all do." It was before the hospital had a suction machine, so he had used a sharp curette. That instrument could have permanently scarred her uterus and made her infertile. We waited fourteen years to have our first child—we were a mess. We could hardly take care of ourselves, let alone a child, and we knew it. We've been married forty-one years and have two children. I waited until two months ago to tell my wife that story.

Being an abortionist means that quite a few of my patients, while they are in stirrups, say, "I don't believe in this, but . . ." or "How can you do this work?" Or "I've always been against this!" Or once, "Are you a real doctor?" And even once, "You better clean those f-cking instruments before you use them on me!" And often they ask, "Will I go to Hell?" The only response I know is, "Do you believe in a forgiving God?"

Being an abortionist means accepting that I'm ending potential human life, but I believe that the rights of present life outweigh the rights of potential life. I hate the term "pro-choice." It sounds like "I'll have vanilla."

I experience a mixture of horror and relief when I crush the skull of a second trimester fetus, knowing that I will be able to safely complete the procedure, but also I will see the squashed face and bulging eyes of the baby I just killed. As the creamy brain tissue pours onto the speculum, I recall what I was told by my ex-chief resident. She still talks to me like I am still her resident. A few years ago, I was visiting her at her clinic, and she said, "Do you see how creamy that brain tissue is? The support structures of the brain don't fully develop until after the first few years of life. That's why shaken baby syndrome is so horrible." I remember the glassy, absent look of one of those babies when I took a tour of a facility for disabled children when I was in medical school.

We have a box in our abortion waiting room labeled "You are not alone." It's where patients can choose to share their thoughts anonymously. This is what one of them wrote: *Dear tiny-tiny baby: I'm sorry to do this to you. I just think you would be so much better off back in the pretty blue sky. Back in the hands of God. I just can't properly take care of you right now. Your brother's only nine* *months old right now. I wish it could be different. It kills me that I have to choose to do this to you: never see you, hear you, hold you . . . just know that I will <u>never</u> forget you. You will <u>always</u> be a part of me!! Love, Mom.*

Being an abortionist means I have two distinct tasks: to be emotionally present and to be technically competent. I have had more advantages than most of my patients. I've had a good education. I've had a good job. After forty-one years, my wife still loves me. But I'm just like them. I've struggled, too. I've made mistakes. We're all doing our best. We're fellow travelers.

Note

1. Partial-Birth Abortion Ban Act of 2003, Pub. L. No. 108-105, 117 Stat. 1201 (2003); 18 U.S.C. § 1531.

Chapter 3

Establishing Abortion Counseling

Terry Beresford

Well, I got into the world of abortion care by accident. I was freelancing, doing a little bit of teacher training, a little bit of miscellaneous consulting of various kinds. And I had a consulting job with the Adlerian Psychology Association of Maryland. I did four sessions of training for these potential group leaders. And at the end of the training, one of the men in the group came up to me and said, "This was very good, and I learned a lot, and my wife has just taken a job as an abortion counselor at the first outpatient abortion clinic in Washington." That was Preterm. "And they've had three different consultants, and they haven't been happy with any of them, and I think you'd be good." So I called them up and said, "I understand you're looking for a consultant to do some training around group work, and I'm available." I knew nothing about abortion. This was in March 1971. Washington, DC, had legalized abortion although there was still an ordinance on the books that said that if you are under eighteen you had to have written consent from a parent or guardian.

I got the world's most wonderful training in group dynamics at Antioch College. I was a student the year Douglas McGregor became college president and brought with him from MIT his sidekick, Irving Knickerbocker. They were right out of the industrial relations training at MIT. My third year in the school, I walked by the bulletin board in the main building. There was this announcement that said, 'The first thirty-two people to sign up here can have a course in group dynamics from Irving Knickerbocker.' I signed my name, and it was a fantastic course. It ended up being two years. It was two full years of dealing with group processes and verbal and nonverbal communication. And it made me know that I wanted to do group work and that I'm good at it. And I had a lot of success. I would get called in to do some organizational development or some training, and there weren't many people doing that in any field, let alone in the field of reproductive health. So I was much in demand for a long time.

I got hired by Preterm and started doing training. Preterm was the first abortion clinic in DC. And it trained people from all over the country when clinics were starting in the early/mid-1970s. When we started Preterm, we ran services starting at 7:30 at night because we had no idea what the complication rate would be, and we didn't want to have to transport patients to the hospital during Washington rush hour. After the first month we discovered we weren't going to have complications, and everything was going fine, and we started doing daytime services. And we ran a morning clinic and an afternoon clinic. On weekdays we did eighty-five procedures a day and on Saturdays 165. And we had doctors on a waiting list who wanted to work for us. How that has changed. These were people who had felt terrible that they hadn't been able to serve their patients when abortion was illegal. Most of them hadn't known where to send somebody or were afraid to do so even if they knew where abortions were being done. And they wanted to make up for what they felt had been their lack. In fact, two of them volunteered their services for free on Saturdays—first-rate doctors. So we were very fortunate.

Here we are. It's 1971. We've just legalized abortion in Washington, DC. Except for New York, there's no other clinic east of the Mississippi. So we're seeing scads of women, many of whom don't even know abortion is legal in DC, have no idea what their issues are, or how complicated it's going to be. At Preterm we felt that every patient should see a counselor alone first. This was partly to assess what the issues were for her, partly to do some birth control counseling, and partly to prepare her adequately for an outpatient procedure which many of them had never had before.

The first five years, before the Right to Life got really organized, we didn't have much trouble, and we learned a lot about patients. And what we learned, I think, was that about 10 percent of the women we saw were badly in need of counseling. They either would not have had an abortion or shouldn't have had one, or they would've had unpleasant after effects from it because they had major issues that they had not yet dealt with and they badly needed a counseling intervention. Usually an hour was enough. Once in a while it took more than that. But those people needed what we offered. About 10 percent of people didn't need a thing. Those were women who already knew a good bit about abortion, didn't have any ambivalence about selecting it for themselves at this particular time, and were pretty well psychologically put together. Some of them said, "I don't want any counseling." Some of them put up with it; some of them were very cooperative, but in general they'd have breezed through psychologically. For the other 80 percent there were some issues. They probably would've made it okay without the counseling, but they were much helped by it. It made the experience not just an okay medical procedure, but it made it a life-changing event for them. We got letters back from people saying what it had meant to them.

Preterm was running group sessions in the waiting room for the boyfriends and parents who had come with abortion patients. I trained their counselors. And they especially wanted help in how to run a good group session with this miscellaneous assortment of people in the waiting room whom they wanted to teach about birth control and also to tell them what was happening to the woman they had brought to the clinic and what an abortion was about and so on. And so that was a sizable part of what I did for them to start with. And then they hired me full time as director of staff development. And I continued to work with their staff for almost two years.

The relationship between female counseling staff and the male doctors at Preterm was very good. Ben Branch, who had been hired as the first medical director for Preterm, was an extraordinary man. He was a Buddhist, and he treated everybody on the staff as equals, including the janitors. He set this tone that there was no hierarchy among the staff, that everybody there was professional and dedicated and got treated that way. In addition, he asked counselors to provide feedback on the doctors: how much pain they caused and what their bedside manner was. Our counselors did an hour's worth of individual counseling with every patient and then accompanied that patient through the procedures. Ben would ask them for feedback about the doctors, and the doctors knew where the feedback was coming from. That setting was a whole different model from what happens in most medical facilities.

We all felt we were on the barricades. We were brand-new stuff, and we were fighting our way, and we were carving it out. I was carving out a model for abortion counseling. These doctors were doing outpatient procedures under local anesthesia, which many doctors had never done before. So everybody had this sense that we were the forefront. So it was like going camping in the rain: hard work, but afterward you thought, "Wasn't that wonderful?" That's what it was like.

I have the world's simplest counseling model. Your task is to help the client explore her feelings and her situation so she can come to some decision and then can take action. That's the model. So what you are exploring is anything that is related to this pregnancy, this abortion, what is happening now with the client. You are not exploring her background, her toilet training. It's situational.

And your responsibility is to help her to the degree that she is willing to be helped, which is to say, some people are not at all [interested] and some people only a limited amount. But if you can, you want her to get to a decision that she is comfortable with. If she can't get there, she goes home. We don't do abortions for people who can't come to a comfortable decision. Comfortable doesn't mean you think it's wonderful; it means that you have acknowledged your ambivalence, and you feel you can handle it. One of the questions you ask people is, "Can you handle it?" And then you facilitate the action by doing, by following up, by whatever the protocol is in the clinic.

I read a lot because what I discovered is that people with formal training in counseling did not have the right kind of training. These were people who were going to make careers out of psychiatric social work, for example. And what they all learned in graduate school was casework. This is not casework. This was short-term crisis intervention counseling. And people weren't getting that kind of training in school. So I hired a lot of lay counselors. In fact, when I hired social workers, which I occasionally did, I used to say, "I'm hiring you in spite of your degree and not because of it." And I read a lot. I read literature on crisis intervention and on basic counseling. I had done graduate work in clinical psych—I'm a grad school dropout. Besides reading, I invented things. For example, when I was at Planned Parenthood, I had access to a very nice audiovisual lab. And I used to ask counselors to role-play certain situations and be videotaped. And then I would study the videotape. And I loved training design. I still get used occasionally by former colleagues and friends who want to take me out to lunch and then pick my brain about some training they have to design. I never did counseling as a profession, although occasionally I would interact with somebody, making clear that I was not a professional counselor.

What I used to teach people was how you do reflecting feelings, how you ask open-ended nonleading, nonloaded questions, how you ask leading questions when you want to bring things down to a conclusion, how you make affirming statements to support the patient. The basic tools of a counselor, that's what I taught people. But beyond that my view was that you can't write an outline for a counseling session. It depends on what the patient comes with, and what she says to start with, and who you are and how you react to what she says. The issue, I always felt, was counselors should not become entrenched. That they had to take time regularly—sometimes with me, sometimes with another counselor, sometimes on their own—to process what had gone on in the session, how they felt about it, and what they thought happened. Where was the turning point? So they were constantly processing their own work. That's what I taught them.

I got fired by Preterm because I stood up to the executive director who did something that I thought was illegal and she fired me. And I once read a wonderful piece that said, "Every successful CEO in the country has been fired at least once." And I went to work for a second abortion clinic called New Woman's Clinic where Ben Branch, who had been medical director for Preterm and also fired by the executive director, worked. When he heard I'd been fired, he called me up and said, "Come to work for us."

Eventually, there were eighteen outpatient services in Washington, DC, and I went to work with Planned Parenthood of Maryland in Baltimore. I worked for them for nine years, first as their director of counseling—they had a major counseling program—and then as the director of their training institute. That training institute had originally been funded by the federal government but was defunded under the Reagan administration. And they moved me into the training to see if I could make a go of it, find money, et cetera. And I did that for about five years, and then I left them. The director of Planned Parenthood was a man named Dan Pelgrom, who now directs Pathfinder. We made a terrific team. He hired me originally because he said there was trouble between the counseling department and the medical department, and he needed someone with my experience to help solve that problem. And I said, "Fine. I'll do it for a year because you're not offering enough pay." But I fell in love with the organization and with the field. And by that time I knew I wanted to stay in the field. I stayed for nine years, and I left when he left the organization, which was already changing some.

Planned Parenthood allowed me an hour and a half every other Monday with counselors to do in-service training, and the counselors got paid for this. I had a little session called "Short Answers to Hard Questions," where we took the kinds of things that a client might raise that would throw you for a minute, but where there is a way to say something brief and short that satisfies. I said to them, "The same stuff comes up from different people over and over and over again. You don't have to re-create a new answer every time. We get an answer that satisfies, and you may use that." But that only pertains to a limited number of things. It doesn't pertain to how you run a counseling session.

When interviewing for counseling positions, I used to ask people two or three questions about abortion. I used to say, "Tell me when you first learned about abortion. How did you learn about it, and what was that like for you?" And I used to ask, "Have you had an abortion yourself?" I would not hire anybody within six months of them having their own abortion because they're still working out their own stuff. And then I used to say, "Tell me any reservations that you have about abortion. We all have some; what are yours?" I was less interested in what they said than in how they reacted. I was always nervous about somebody who said, "I don't have any trouble with abortion in any way." I would also ask, "What kind of patient do you think would give you the most trouble?" And I wouldn't hire somebody who said, "Nobody. Nobody would give me trouble. I'm comfortable with everybody." Bullshit! So I'm looking for people who have some sense of self-awareness and some sense of process. That's the key stuff. And people who haven't recently had an abortion themselves and who seem to be well put together. At Maryland, I had a counseling staff that ranged in age from twenty-one to sixty-eight. I had no requirements except that they came across in the interview as able to conduct themselves as an adult.

I went back to Preterm as their executive director because Preterm wanted to go out of business. For a variety of reasons, the board of directors was tired and wanted to close down shop. They hired me to come in and be their last executive director and help them go out of business clean. I engineered a take-over by Planned Parenthood of Washington, DC. We sold our assets to Planned Parenthood, went out of business clean—paying off all obligations including all staff obligations—and I made the agreement with them that they would pick up the existing Preterm staff who had years of experience and give them a chance, with the exception of a couple of administrative people.

In the early 1980s, the National Right to Life held their annual convention in Washington, DC. I was the director of Preterm then, and I got a phone call from the National Organization for Women. They always have spies at Right to Life conventions. They said, "One of our spies said they're planning a massive attack on a clinic tomorrow morning." That would've been a Saturday morning. "They've described the outside of the clinic. We think it's you." At that point, Preterm was housed in a three-story row house at 17th and Q Street. I got the staff together, and I said to them, "We've had word that the Right to Life will demonstrate in front of the clinic tomorrow morning and that they have planted an appointment to get somebody inside the clinic." So I said to Faith, who was the person who made appointments, "If I told you that there was somebody who was a plant from the Right to Life for tomorrow, could you make a guess as to who it might be?" She said, "Oh sure." She had this list of appointments. She said, "Well, it's not any of these people because they're all referred by Group Health, and none of them, nobody would risk their connection to their HMO provider. So it's not one of them. These people have all had . . . have been here before or have had a previous abortion. It's not them." And she says, "It's probably one of these two."

One of them was a young woman, Faith said, very well spoken, who refused to give any information over the phone. We didn't ask for much, but we did ask

if they were under the care of a psychiatrist because we had them bring the letter if they were. And she said, "She wouldn't give any information, and that's
puzzling. Then this one," she said, "this is another strange one. This girl asked
for a 7:30 A.M. appointment." That's when we started on Saturdays. Now most
people don't want to come at 7:30 in the morning—most people don't even know
we start that early. "And she, when I told her that the 7:30 appointments were
all taken, she could come at 10:30. She said, well, her boyfriend would drop
her off at 7:30, and she would just wait." Patients don't do that. Nobody goes
three hours early for their appointment.

We had thirty-six appointments for that day, and we tried to call all those
women to warn them and to give them a chance to reschedule, and some of them
we didn't reach. One of them was as policewoman who said she was going to
reschedule; she didn't want to meet her buddies on the street. But eighteen
women said, "We're coming," and they did. So then I said, "Who's the physician operating tomorrow?" Somebody said, "It's Mark Jerome." He was our clinic
director, a wonderful Haitian man who could do an abortion so the woman
didn't feel a thing. So we called him and said, "Do you want to work tomorrow?" He said, "Certainly, it's my job. But I'm coming in the back door." And
then I said to the staff, "Anybody who doesn't want to come to work tomorrow
doesn't have to." Everybody said, "We're coming."

So at 7:30 in the morning there are 250 Right to Lifers amassed in front of
the building. Joe Scheidler is there in his dirty white suit with his bullhorn
shouting at me on the porch: "It takes a Jew like you to run a place like this."[1]
You know that story. My director of counseling is a gay man who is six-foot-
five, and he's standing with me on the porch. There are six policemen. And
I said to the police captain, "I want you to clear a path so that patients and staff
can get in." He said, "Ma'am, this is an ugly crowd, and I don't have enough
police. After rush hour is over, the precincts will free up some other men. In
the meantime, we'll just lift people over the heads of the protestors and up onto
your porch." So that's what they started doing. It was incredible. This was a day
to remember.

Pretty soon this young girl comes up. She's wearing white duck pants and
a white duck jacket, and she has spiked hair, half-black, half-blonde. And I said,
"I need to see your ID and the letter from your doctor." She had said on the
phone that she was epileptic. She said, "Well, I, I, I, don't have any of that
because when I was pushing my way through that crowd, somebody stole my
purse." And I knew that that was the plant because those protestors, as ugly as
they are, they are not into purse snatching. I just knew this had to be her. I said
to her, "Look, I'm sorry. You're going to have to have your ID and your money

and the letter from your doctor, or we're not going to be able to do your abortion." She said, "Well, you have to because they told me on the phone that I was borderline and I needed to come in today or it would be too late." I said, "Well, what we'll do is make a referral for you for next Monday for Washington Hospital Center where you can have a later term abortion." She said, "Well, I'll give you the name of my doctor, and you can call him." I said, "I'm sorry, but my medical director would not find that acceptable. We have no idea who we're talking to." She said, "You know who I am, don't you?" I said, "Yes, I do." She opens up her jacket, and she's wearing a T-shirt that says, "I'm pro-life." So I had her removed from the porch.

Meantime, there are two postscripts to this story. We had a counselor meeting with every patient as she came in. Even before we did lab work or anything, we took them into a room and debriefed from their ugly experience out on the street. And then we started doing procedures. After about an hour, it occurred to me I didn't want the patients leaving out the front door and pushing their way back through that crowd. So I took the police captain aside, and I said, "Look. I have a back door to this clinic that leads out into a back alley. But I want police protection out there so we can have patients leave that way." He said, "Oh, we'll do better than that. We'll bring the paddy wagon right up the alley, and they can get right into the paddy wagon, and we will drive them several blocks away and let them out far away from the crowd." And I said, "Fine. Will you take their boyfriends and their mothers in the paddy wagon also?" He said, "Certainly."

So I sent one of the counselors in the recovery room, and there were three women ready to leave: the first three women, a Black woman who was a teacher in a DC public school system, and two younger women. And the counselor said to them, "You can leave now, and I'm going to escort you out the back door where the police will provide you protection." And this teacher stood up, and she said, "I'm not going out the back door—never again." And these other two women said, "Well, I guess we have to go with her, don't we?" The three of them hooked arms and walked out the front door. So we got through the day, and indeed, after rush hour was over, more police came, and they cleared a pathway, and eventually the protestors went away.

Anyway, the end of the day comes. It's about 3:30 in the afternoon; the patients are all gone, and most of the staff are gone. There are a few of us left, and we're putting away the files and cleaning up, and there's a knock on the door. And there's a teenager and her boyfriend standing there, and I said, "Honey, I'm awfully sorry, but we're closed." She said, "I know, but I just have to speak to you for a minute." I said, "Okay, what's on your mind?" She said, "Well, my boyfriend and I were walking by here this morning, and we saw all those people there, and I said to him, 'You know, that's not right what they're doing. They shouldn't do that.' He said, 'Well, what are you going to do about it?' And it's been on my mind all day, and it bothered me. I, we're on our way home, but I thought I would just ask you this question: Do you take money?" So, I said, "Would you like to make a contribution to our abortion loan fund?" She said, "Yes," and she wrote a check for thirty dollars, handed me the check, turned to her boyfriend and said, "I feel a lot better now."

I was invited to come to the 1975 conference in Knoxville, Tennessee, to do a workshop on counseling. I had just started work for Planned Parenthood. There were two doctors and a lawyer who chose to attend the counseling workshop. The two doctors were Phil Darney and Curtis Boyd. And the lawyer was Roy Lucas. Frances [Kissling] was at that meeting as were Penny Steenblock and other people. And so about ten of us met at the end of the conference; we met together and talked about the need to set up a national organization. That group first became NAAF [National Association of Abortion Facilities]. I had nothing to do with them. Frances Kissling's group was first called the National Abortion Council and then NAF [National Abortion Federation] and that was my connection.[2]

That board of directors—who would think of putting together such a disparate group of people? You had Planned Parenthood and the for-profits and the not-for-profits and the private doctors and the Feminist Health Coalition, who made trouble at every turn. The board meetings were a nightmare. There were always issues. First, the question of standards. The factions divided between those who went to NAF to set standards and uphold them and against the people, feminists particularly, who worried about access to services and argued that you didn't want to deny people a chance to go to a clinic who might not meet all the standards right away, et cetera. And the cost of enforcing standards was an issue for NAF.

Part of the issue for any organization that is set up the way NAF is, is that people's primary loyalty is to their own organization back home. It takes time to develop loyalty to this new federation. It becomes easier to accept the compromise when you get to know people well and when you begin to have something vested in the organization. As that began to develop, people had more tolerance for one another and more devotion to wanting to see the organization succeed.

Today, most clinics are not doing what I would call counseling. They're doing informed consent, but they're not doing counseling. Over time, I think, the counseling changed. We needed a better evaluation of patient needs. Many places found that if they knew how to train their counselors to do evaluations, which is the hardest job that the counselor does, they could cut down on counseling time and perhaps let some people by with just informed consent. The trouble was that most places were not giving their counselors that kind of training; and doing an evaluation in a short amount of time before surgery is a very difficult task. That got combined with financial constraints. Education and counseling are always cut out of everybody's budget. So that's where they cut back. Some clinics just did away with counseling altogether and trained their nurses to do a decent job of informed consent. Hardly anybody that I know of is still doing counseling. Many went to what they called group counseling, but it wasn't really group counseling: it was group informed consent with an occasional question—Does anybody want to see a counselor or talk to the nurse privately? The quality of that varied according to who was doing it, and what kind of training they'd had, and how much time they were given, et cetera.

So that all shifted over time. When I was doing counselor training for NAF, we had a lot of people attending those counseling sessions, including some clinic managers who wanted to know more about counseling, and wanted to see how they could train their own staff better, and so on. But that also changed. I don't know at what point, because at some point I stopped doing it for NAF.

Notes

1. In the 1980s and 1990s, Joseph M. Scheidler was known for traveling around the country to appear at local antiabortion pickets where he drew crowds of protestors. He was also very active developing antiabortion protest and legal strategies. Scheidler is the author of the 1985 book *Closed: 99 Ways to Stop Abortion* (Rockford, IL: Tan Books), which sets out many of his strategies.

2. Frances Kissling was the first president of NAF. She started her work in abortion care in 1970, when she became the director of the Pelham Medical Group in Westchester, New York, one of the first freestanding abortion clinics in New York. She went on to become the president of Catholics for Choice, a position she held from 1982 to 2007.

Part 2

Clinics

The model of the freestanding abortion clinic appealed not only to physicians like Dr. Morris Turner and Dr. Marc Heller. It also offered feminists seeking an alternative to traditional medical care the opportunity to imagine health care services that put women's needs at the center. Most physicians were unresponsive to women's health care needs and unwilling to answer their questions or address their concerns.

Women's frustration with the medical profession stood out most clearly in their relationships with their obstetricians and gynecologists, most of whom were male. As the specialists responsible for women's most intimate health care needs, ob-gyns also functioned as gatekeepers when women sought access to birth control and abortion.[1] Starting in the late 1960s, women across the country began to challenge the patriarchal attitude of medical professionals. Their physicians, they complained, were "condescending, paternalistic, judgmental, and non-informative."[2] A group of women in Boston came together to discuss their health care providers and search for answers to their medical questions. Group members researched and educated one another on topics related to childbirth, sexuality, and reproduction. In December 1970 they published the results under the title *Women and Their Bodies*, which three years later became better known as *Our Bodies, Ourselves*.[3]

When the United States Supreme Court legalized abortion on January 22, 1973, women across the country quickly grasped the enormous implications that the decision could hold for women's health care. Twenty-one-year-old office assistant Renee Chelian, whose essay in this section reflects on the difficulties maintaining a feminist practice in the context of antiabortion politics today,

immediately began to schedule abortion patients for Dr. Gilbert Higuera in his
Highland Park, Michigan, office. Prior to the *Roe v. Wade* decision, Chelian and
Higuera had flown every weekend to Buffalo, New York, where abortion had
been legal since 1970. There, they had provided abortion services out of a small
office. Now Higuera closed his Buffalo clinic and moved all the equipment into
his regular ob-gyn office outside Detroit. "For me, everything changed," Chelian remembered. "All of a sudden, I had a dream about what I thought things
should be like."[4]

Feminists hoped that the legalization of abortion would not only make
abortion safe and accessible but also change medical practice. When Chelian
thought of the early legal abortions Dr. Higuera had performed in his small
Buffalo clinic, she thought of them as an act of compassion. After *Roe*, she hoped
that Higuera would improve the conditions under which he offered legal abortions. Indeed, across the country, feminists tried to influence the establishment
of abortion services. While physicians, most of them male, sought to keep tight
control over the medical aspects of abortion care, they employed women as
nurses, counselors, office assistants, and clinic administrators. Many of these
women brought their ideas about women-friendly health care services into the
newly established abortion clinics.[5]

Inspired by the emerging women's health movement and frustrated with traditional medical care, women looked to the field of abortion care as an opportunity to shape a more feminist future in medicine. The model of the freestanding
abortion clinic offered feminists seeking an alternative to traditional medical
care the opportunity to put their vision of woman-centered health care into practice. Many saw women's access to affordable abortions as central to women's
self-determination. Across the country, women opened women's health clinics,
some of which integrated abortion services as a logical extension of feminist
health care. Carol Downer, a California housewife turned women's health activist, established a group of clinics, the Feminist Women's Health Centers (FWHC).
Intrigued by Downer's vision, feminists in Michigan, New Hampshire, Florida,
and Georgia opened clinics affiliated with the FWHC in Detroit, Concord, Tal-
lahassee, and Atlanta, respectively. In other states, Vermont, Massachusetts, and
Iowa, feminists followed suit with clinics that were not affiliated with the
FWHC.[6]

Feminist clinics embedded abortion services into a comprehensive program
of health education, geared at transforming patient consciousness. Offering free
information over the phone was part of a democratization process geared at empowering patients. "People were calling us all day long to ask the simplest
questions," Chelian remembered. "How do you put on a condom? And how do

you know if you have crabs or lice? . . . It was basic information that they had never been able to get . . . anywhere else."[7]

Feminist clinics also sought to offer written educational materials, complete with images that did not depict all female bodies as pregnant. But finding a drawing of a cervix or of an empty uterus was a challenging task. Chelian finally located a booklet with appropriate images from the Montreal Health Press that she began to hand out to patients. Others set out to write their own educational materials, ranging from short pamphlets to educational treatises that included in-depth discussions of a number of health issues.[8]

Clinics also began to offer free pregnancy testing and free samples of birth control pills. This proved revolutionary for women's ability to control their reproduction. Steeped in the women's health movement, activists sought to educate patients about their bodies and encourage them to make their own choices.[9] "We all felt we were living through some giant change," Chelian commented. "We were seeing women who were experiencing for the first time in their lives the opportunity to have control over their reproductive lives."[10]

Equally important to feminist clinics was the delivery of services by women rather than men. Feminists hoped that if patients experienced services delivered by women, this would trigger a sense of empowerment for patients. It would finally allow women to make their own informed choices regarding reproductive health care and ideally lead patients themselves to question traditional gender roles.

Women who worked in feminist collectives retained ultimate control over the clinic. They could thus debate these issues and determine how to structure patient services. Women like Chelian, who worked in abortion clinics owned by men, however, found that prompting change was much more difficult. Chelian recalls arguing with Dr. Higuera about answering patient questions over the phone. The integration of abortion into ob-gyn services itself, feminists realized, would not lead to a change in the hierarchical relationship between physicians as the arbiters of basic information of sexual health and patients in need of health education. "There wasn't going to be any evolution or any changing with him," Chelian concluded about her work with Dr. Higuera.[11]

Nevertheless, physicians and businessmen who opened and invested in the new abortion services provided important financial and institutional backing for an emerging network of abortion clinics. And in the best of cases they offered women like Renee Chelian the opportunity to help shape women's health services. Indeed, Chelian's story clearly illustrates this. Only two months after the legalization of abortion, she decided to leave her position with Dr. Higuera and began to work for Lenn Sands. Sands had opened an abortion clinic in

Detroit—the third in the city. In addition, he opened two more clinics in Dallas, Texas, and Metairie, Louisiana, just outside New Orleans. He put Chelian in charge of the Detroit clinic.

Chelian quickly discovered that decisions were hers to make. "The first time I called him up with a problem, he said, 'I don't know, darling. How do you think you should handle that?' And he hung up on me. . . . [That] was when I realized, 'Oh my God, the buck stops with me. I'm in charge, and he's not going to help me.' So it was a huge growth step for me because what I did realize was I could figure it out."[12] In 1976, Chelian opened her own clinic, Northland Family Planning.

Chelian's story is not unusual. Indeed, women across the country realized that they could "figure it out." The opportunities provided in the early clinics offered a generation of women an avenue into the medical field—not only as medical staff but also as counselors, health administrators, and clinic directors. Once in those positions, women could participate in the shaping of more feminist and woman-centered clinics. At the annual meetings of the National Abortion Federation, women clinic owners met each other. They compared experiences, gave each other advice, and formed a community of independent clinic owners intent on providing the best woman-centered care possible. "We were starting to connect with other providers," Chelian remembers. "We were starting to learn from each other. We weren't functioning as a doctor's office anymore. It wasn't the doctor comes in and tells everybody what to do."[13]

Independent clinics like Chelian's functioned as innovators in the field of abortion care. Flexible in their service delivery and without a male boss or larger organization to whom they were accountable, the women who opened independent clinics were able to forge new solutions in health care delivery. "We were the first places in the country doing outpatient surgery really," Chelian explained. "I noticed that there were a lot of patients the doctors were turning away. They wanted to get medical clearance for somebody who had asthma, and when I would say, 'All right, so how do we take care of these patients?' And then it would be, 'All right, well, we need to have a protocol that if they're asthmatic, they have to bring their inhaler with them, but we need to keep an inhaler in the crash cart.' Okay, and we would make a protocol."[14] Determined to increase the safety of abortion procedures and expand services to as many women as possible, independent clinics were at the forefront of research and innovation, adapting procedures and trying new services.

The autonomy that made independent clinics so flexible, however, also made them particularly vulnerable to antiabortion laws and regulations. Since the 1970s, many cities and townships had relied on local ordinances, building codes, and zoning restrictions to prevent the opening of abortion clinics. Following the 1993 decision in *Planned Parenthood v. Casey*, states began to pass antiabortion regulations that targeted specifically abortion clinics and that went beyond what was necessary to ensure patient safety. Legislators passed these so-called TRAP [targeted regulation of abortion providers] laws under the guise that they would make abortion services safer, although their primary purpose has always been to limit access to abortion. None of the restrictions increased the safety of abortion procedures, which were already the safest outpatient procedures available.

Most TRAP laws apply a state's standard for ambulatory surgical centers (ASCs) to abortion clinics, even though surgical centers tend to provide riskier, more invasive procedures and use higher levels of sedation. TRAP regulations often include requirements that may necessitate relocation or costly changes to a clinic's physical layout and structure. They set standards that are intended to be difficult, if not impossible to meet, forcing the facilities unable to comply out of business. In 2016, the U.S. Supreme Court struck down two of the most burdensome TRAP laws that had been passed in Texas: a regulation that required physicians to have hospital-admitting privileges at a local hospital and requirements that Texas abortion facilities meet the state standard for ASCs. As Amy Hagstrom Miller explains in her essay, these regulations would have had a devastating impact on the experiences of both providing and receiving abortion care. They also would have forced the closure of most clinics.

Both essays in this section ponder the question, How can clinics operating on the defensive against overregulation and harassment by state health officials provide feminist care that is patient centered and offer an environment that is both physically and emotionally warm and supportive? If antiabortion legislation has done one thing, it has made it difficult and at times impossible for abortion providers to do what feminist clinics originally set out to do: provide women with a health care environment that feels warm, secure, and supportive.

Notes

1. Johanna Schoen, *Abortion after Roe* (Chapel Hill: University of North Carolina Press, 2015), 5–6.
2. Boston Women's Health Collective, 1973, 1, as quoted in Sandra Morgen, *Into Our Own Hands: The Women's Health Movement in the United States, 1969–1990* (New Brunswick, NJ: Rutgers University Press, 2002), 4.
3. Wendy Kline, *Bodies of Knowledge: Sexuality, Reproduction, and Women's Health in the Second Wave* (Chicago: University of Chicago Press, 2010); Kathy Davis, *The Making of "Our Bodies, Ourselves": How Feminism Travels across Borders* (Durham, NC: Duke University Press, 2007).
4. Renee Chelian, interview with Peg Johnston, 2008.

5. Carole E. Joffe, Tracy A. Weitz, and C. L. Stacey, "Uneasy Allies: Pro-Choice Physicians, Feminist Health Activists, and the Struggle for Abortion Rights," *Sociology of Health and Illness* 26, no. 6 (2004): 775–796, https://doi.org/10.1111/j.0141-9889 .2004.00418.x.

6. Schoen, *Abortion after Roe*, 42; Morgen, *Into Our Own Hands*; Anne Enke, *Finding the Movement: Sexuality, Contested Space, and Feminist Activism* (Durham, NC: Duke University Press, 2007); Wendy Simonds, *Abortion at Work: Ideology and Practice in a Feminist Clinic* (New Brunswick, NJ: Rutgers University Press, 1996).

7. Chelian, interview with Johnston, 2008.

8. *Our Bodies, Ourselves* from the Boston Women's Health Collective was first published as a newsprint pamphlet in 1970; it included chapters on anatomy and physiology, sexuality, myths about women, venereal disease, birth control, and other topics. The first edition in 1970 had 130 pages; by 2005 it had grown to an 832-page reference work. Many college campuses came up with their own publications on sexuality, reproduction, and sexual health.

9. Pattie Pressley, interviewed by LeAnn Erickson, undated [ca. 1993], Emma Goldman Clinic Papers, Iowa Women's Archive, University of Iowa Libraries, Iowa City, IA.

10. Chelian, interview with Johnston, 2008.

11. Chelian, interview with Johnston, 2008.

12. Renee Chelian, interview with Johanna Schoen, March 11, 2011, Sterling Heights, MI.

13. Chelian, interview with Schoen, March 11, 2011.

14. Chelian, interview with Schoen, March 11, 2011. See also Schoen, *Abortion after Roe*, esp. chapters 1 and 3.

Chapter 4

Providing Compassionate Abortion Care in a Hostile Climate

Amy Hagstrom Miller

Adapt, pivot, adjust, challenge. These four words are something Whole Woman's Health and other abortion providers know how to do all too well. We adapt quickly to policy changes, we pivot when new regulations are placed on us, we adjust when lawmakers pass new antiabortion laws that further restrict how we provide care, and often we have to challenge those new laws in court.

Whole Woman's Health currently manages eight abortion clinics in five states: Texas, Virginia, Maryland, Minnesota, and Indiana. Because we operate in both "red" and "blue" states, we work in what often feels like two different Americas. We are committed to raising the standard of care and maintaining access to quality abortion care in communities throughout the South and the Midwest of the United States, areas with the most restrictive laws and regulations on abortion care. Since our founding in 2003, we have acquired fourteen existing independent clinics and started three new ones across the country. We have also merged three clinics, closed six, and reopened one. And there have been countless renovations, moves, and construction projects along the way. We do all of this in order to provide holistic, woman-centered care with the compassion, respect, and dignity that all people deserve.

Over the past decades, the hyperregulation and layers of laws targeting abortion clinics [targeted regulation of abortion providers, or TRAP, laws] have contributed to significant changes in how abortion care is provided and received in America. Stringent abortion regulations have influenced our field tremendously. The regulatory environment has changed our daily work and our relationships with our patients. And it has fundamentally changed how people experience the service of abortion care in the United States. In fact, there is a generation of people who now expect regulatory barriers to abortion—unnecessary restrictions have been normalized.

Some of the realities of the hostile climate that abortion providers and patients face are obvious. Among those have been regulations requiring that abortion clinics meet the standards of ambulatory surgery centers (ASCs), requirements that abortion providers have admitting privileges at a local hospital, mandatory delays/waiting periods, bans that prohibit abortions after 20 weeks' gestation, state-mandated "informed consent," forced ultrasounds, and state licensing and inspections. Less obvious but also hostile to the provision of abortion care are Medicaid funding bans, insurance bans, no coverage for family planning, and a lack of sex education. Nearly invisible is the use of state power to harass and intimidate abortion providers through inspections, fines, hearings, and the random and inconsistent enforcement of regulations. Similarly, the internalized stigma patients and abortion providers endure, often feeling like outsiders, combined with the internalized oppression that accompanies abortion care for those who provide and those who receive the care also contribute on a deep and nearly immeasurable level to a hostile climate. And finally, and most cruelly shocking, are the attempts by state lawmakers to take advantage of the public health crisis created by COVID-19 to try to ban all abortions as nonessential health care.

In 2013, Texas passed a series of restrictions on abortion clinics that included the requirement that abortion providers have admitting privileges at a hospital within thirty miles of the clinic and that clinics meet the same standards as ASCs. Indeed, state legislators passed similar laws in twenty states.[1] Meeting ASC standards meant that clinic owners would need to renovate their building, increase safety, modify parking, and increase staffing levels to meet the standards of a hospital room. These standards were not supported by medical data and did not advance health and safety. Rather, they were political in nature, designed to shutter clinics and thereby ban abortion. The environmental changes necessitated by the new restrictions determined the width of clinic hallways, forbade any artwork on the walls, and would have resulted in a building where the walls are white and the atmosphere cold. By contrast with Whole Woman's Health examination rooms, the surgical suite of an ASC is giant and intimidating (Figures 4.1 and 4.2). Staff in an ASC are unable to offer patients warm tea or provide them with fleece blankets in recovery; instead, all patients are completely undressed and clad in standard tissue gowns. As a result, the patients are not only freezing, but also lose their individuality and identity. Staff, in turn, are required to wear personal protective equipment intended for surgical operations that creates a literal barrier to their connection with patients (Figures 4.3 and 4.4). In addition, the operating

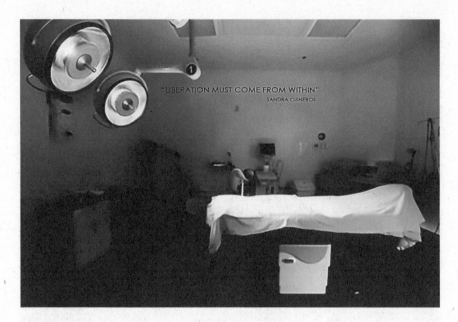

Figure 4.1 Ambulatory surgery center operating room

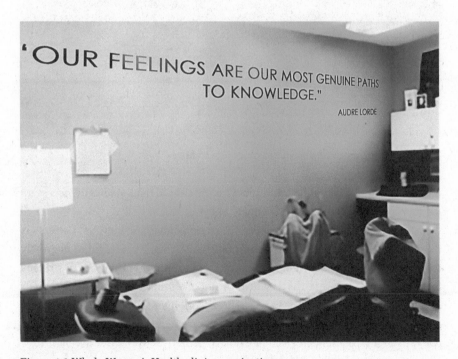

Figure 4.2 Whole Woman's Health clinic examination room

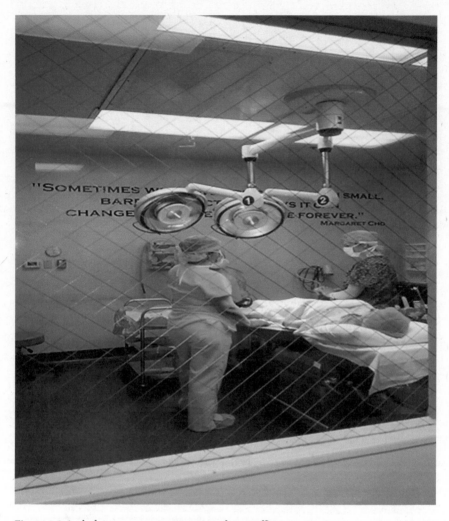

Figure 4.3 Ambulatory surgery center procedure staffing

room is required to be staffed with many more people than medically necessary for abortion care, increasing the patients' sense of vulnerability.

Building community and opportunities for connection between patients is the most important factor in reducing abortion stigma. Hyperregulation greatly reduces opportunities for connection and community. Patients have privacy forced on them, whether they want it or not. Curtains between aftercare beds divide the patients and leave them isolated. State-mandated information can no longer be offered in a group setting where women might connect with each other, react to the information, and ask questions together. Instead, information is now given one on one with the physician.

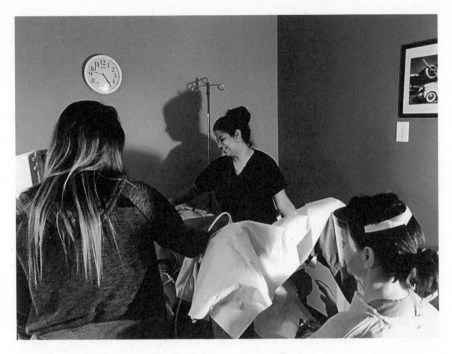

Figure 4.4 Whole Woman's Health clinic procedure staffing

Much of the hostile environment is nearly invisible to the public, but it is extremely powerful for staff and patients. Instead of being the patient's advocate, laws regulating abortion clinics today put us in the position of enforcer and restrictor. This is difficult for our staff, who went into this line of work to help people from a deep commitment to human rights and justice. Now we find ourselves forced to educate women about restrictions we do not agree with and enforce state regulations 24/7 that are completely unnecessary. In fact, we have become agents of the state—forced to provide our patients with propaganda not rooted in science. The patients' trust in us is understandably diminished, and the staff begin to second-guess themselves. As the staff experience hostile inspection after inspection, they start to wonder if we are doing something wrong, if the services we provide lie outside "normal medicine," if they are qualified to work in our clinic. And patients begin to think that maybe abortion is complicated and risky. They worry that maybe they won't be safe. Of course, nothing could be further from the truth: abortion remains one of the safest procedures in medicine.

A high percentage of staff work time is spent on complying with and managing state regulations. The staff are required to draft protocols, prepare for inspections, attend and respond to inspections, and write plans of care. The number of required logs to record data is overwhelming as is the number of agencies we are forced to comply with: local departments of health, the Centers for Medicare & Medicaid Services, pharmacy boards, nursing boards, medical boards, environmental quality commissions, insurance companies, the Joint Commission on Accreditation of Healthcare Organization, and the Accreditation Association for Ambulatory Healthcare.

For most of these regulations the inspection processes connected to them are not rooted in health and safety or scientific facts, nor are they about abortion safety outcomes. The oversight is excessive for an in-office procedure like abortion, which includes no incisions or actual surgery. The regulations are designed, rather, for political purposes—to disrupt, distract, delay, and intimidate. As a result, our patients' abortion experiences have changed dramatically. It is now a medical experience that is often complex, scary, and serious. In addition, the patients' experience of us as health care workers has changed as well. We have become the enforcer of laws, the presenter of barriers. And we have become wholly clinical; we no longer can establish a personal relationship with the patients rooted in compassion, advocacy, and support.

Finally, *our* experience of the work changes as well. There is less depth, less ability to connect with the patients and other staff. There is no time for informal chitchat and the connections made through that. The stress in the workplace increases because the staff are now working in a "gotcha" environment.

It is important to note that restrictions that cause delay or that regulate hallway width and examination room size, for example, do not make abortion safer. There was no safety problem with abortion care in the first place. Our safety record with our patients and the outcomes of our care are the same in states with minimal regulatory interference (Minnesota and Maryland) as they are in states with hyperregulation (Texas and Indiana). In fact, hyperregulation has been tied to making abortion less safe. The increased driving time related to clinic closures and two-visit requirements—often more than 150 miles each way—as well as the mandatory delays and insurance bans to affordability can push people into the second trimester. These are all barriers that increase risks.[2]

In 2013, Whole Woman's Health filed two lawsuits challenging both the requirement that abortion providers have admitting privileges and that clinics meet ASC requirements. When the admitting privileges requirement took effect, the number of abortion clinics in Texas dropped from forty-four to eighteen. The courts suspended the enforcement of the ASC regulations in November 2013 as the case wound its way through the courts. Had the ASC regulations gone into full effect, the number of clinics offering abortion services in Texas would have dropped to five.

On June 27, 2016, the U.S. Supreme Court ruled by a 5–3 vote in *Whole Woman's Health v. Hellerstedt* that Texas cannot place restrictions on the delivery of abortion services that create an undue burden for women seeking an abortion unless those restrictions advance women's health and safety and those claims can be supported by scientific evidence.[3] The court struck down key provisions of the law—requiring doctors who perform abortions to have difficult-to-obtain "admitting privileges" at a local hospital and requiring clinics to have costly hospital-grade facilities—as violating a woman's right to an abortion. These provisions, the majority concluded, do not offer medical benefits sufficient to justify the burdens on access that each imposes. "Each places a substantial obstacle in the path of women seeking a pre-viability abortion, each constitutes an undue burden on abortion access, and each violates the federal Constitution."[4]

The global health pandemic surrounding COVID-19 exposes how quickly and to what extent antiabortion politicians and activists were willing to exploit the moment to effectively ban abortion. In March 2020, Texas Governor Greg Abbott issued a statewide order limiting "nonessential" medical procedures to "curb the use of medical supplies hospitals will need as they prepare for escalating infections." He was referring to personal protective equipment (PPE). Governor Abbott included abortion in the list of medical services deemed nonessential, in effect banning the procedure in Texas for twenty out of thirty days in March and April 2020.

Even in states where governors deemed abortions exempt from "nonessential or elective" procedures, abortion services were not necessarily safe. In Minnesota, for instance, Governor Tim Waltz's order deemed abortion care essential procedures, which allowed clinics to continue to operate. In April, however, several right-wing organizations and medical providers seeking to block abortions in Minnesota during the coronavirus pandemic challenged the governor's order, suing Minnesota Governor Tim Waltz and the five abortion providers in the state. This lawsuit was just another attempt to restrict abortion care under the guise of health and safety.

We know that abortion is time sensitive and cannot be delayed. In this pandemic, people are losing their jobs, health care coverage, childcare services, and much more. In an era with such great uncertainty, the need for safe, timely, and compassionate abortion services is even more apparent. Multiple organizations, including the World Health Organization and the American College of Obstetricians and Gynecologists, have classified abortion as essential health care, and medical research has shown that extreme abortion restrictions do not stop women from getting abortions—they stop women from receiving safe abortions. This could increase unnecessary emergency department visits, infections, infertility, and possible death. These restrictions create health care disparities that show up even more starkly in this pandemic. And that impact is felt most deeply by the uninsured, those who live in rural communities, and by young people and people of color.

The effects on pregnant women are devastating. In Texas, hundreds of women were denied essential abortion care services for nearly a month while we fought Governor Abbott's order in court. Going round after round with the state made for a month that gave us, and our patients, whiplash. We were forced to cancel hundreds of appointments on multiple occasions, hearing pleas of desperation from patients who begged us to see them. Our staff were once again put in a terrible position by the state and were forced to enforce restrictions that went against their beliefs and against science. The executive order forced many patients to continue pregnancies against their will; they had to just wait to see if their rights would be restored. Some patients were able to travel out of state by car, even during this pandemic, to receive the care they deserved. With financial help from our abortion fund, we even helped some who were coming up on the legal limit fly out of state to clinics in Charlottesville and Baltimore managed by Whole Woman's Health. Most women, however, had to just wait, adding even more uncertainty to their lives during this pandemic.

The month-long stunt by Texas leaders was never about keeping Texans healthy or preserving PPE. It was about pushing their antiabortion agenda and controlling what women can and cannot do with their own bodies. If they truly had concern for health care outcomes during COVID-19 they would have allowed abortion providers to practice telemedicine and nixed the two-visit requirement and mandatory delays for patients seeking abortion services.

On top of this opposition from antiabortion forces, often strengthened through the power of the state, we abortion providers also must deal with abortion stigma from inside the progressive movement. Many progressives and movement leaders do not talk about actual abortion care unless they must. Abortion is not framed as a moral good but as a solution to a problem. Often this means that their talk in defense of abortion care is reactionary. Pro-choice leaders on "our side" are often afraid of what abortion providers might say. Many of them have never been to an abortion clinic, seen a procedure, or worked with those of us who provide the care. Providers are often shushed or kept out of the inner loop of movement strategy.

Funding and support focus on advocacy, communications, or policy, not on the actual provision of services. Allies are often uncomfortable talking about the complexities of abortion openly and honestly. They are also not well-versed in abortion provision. They frequently do not understand the regulations in place or the impact the regulations have on clinics and patients.

And in our movement people often struggle with how to talk about the tough issues regarding abortion, issues that lie beyond the rhetoric of rights and health. Antiabortion activists seize on this! *They* talk a lot about abortion and abortion providers. They talk about twenty-week bans, discuss fetal pain, and frame proposals for ASCs and physicians' hospital privileges as safety concerns. They argue that abortion providers are money-grubbing profiteers and discuss funding bans. They argue against sex selection in abortion, even co-opting a feminist angle. And they claim that abortion is Black genocide.

Abortion is messy—literally and figuratively. It is complex. No one gets pregnant in order to have an abortion. The experience is not on anyone's bucket list. In fact, no one wants to be our customer. In the services realm, we deal with the things many folks do not want to talk about—blood, tissue, money, cramping, grief. To us providers, the work is not abstract—it is not a "choice" and it is not "access." Pro-choice allies often tend to deflect the issue of abortion care. "You offer other services, right?" they ask us. "You don't just do abortions?" "I mean, you do birth control and pap smears, right?" Or they note any of the following: "Abortion should be rare," "Abortion is a tragedy," "Most later term abortions are fetal anomalies," and "We should compromise on abortions in cases of rape and incest." They demand and apologize: "Abortion is only 3 percent of what we do," or "I am pro-choice, but I'd never have an abortion." And they say, "I don't believe in abortion as birth control," "I am not the kind of woman who would have an abortion," and "Christian women don't have abortions."

Our allies may often be afraid of what the providers will say, but our patients are not afraid. They ask us all the questions, and we talk about it all with them. We are open and honest. There are no secrets here.

The clinics where these conversations are most likely to happen are the classic independent feminist clinics owned or operated by women and human rights supporters. These are also the clinics that are closing at a faster rate than the clinics owned by physicians or Planned Parenthood. Currently, there are still several independent feminist clinics open: Whole Woman's Health, Northland Family Planning, the Women's Centers, the Emma Goldman Clinic, Preterm, the Cedar River Clinics, the Feminist Women's Health Center in Atlanta, to name a few. We are the providers who entered the field through the human rights, justice, and feminist lens. Advocacy is at the core of why we are providers. The medicine and the business aspects of running a clinic are important, but they are not our purpose. We engage. Advocacy and abortion provision go hand in hand for us.

Is the independent clinic care model obsolete? Are we outdated in the services we provide? Or are we being targeted because of our patient-centered advocacy? Are we intentionally being replaced by high volume, sterile, safe, "uterus emptiers"? Is this progress? Normalization? Mainstreaming? Or is this a deliberate chipping away at the core of a specialty that is patient centered and holistic by its very nature?

Independent providers need to open our clinic doors and step out into the "movement," to engage in the conversation about abortion in this county, and to destigmatize abortion and abortion providers. We cannot hide in the shadows; we must come into the light. We *know* how to talk about abortion in ways that will shift the stigma that allows for the passage of antiabortion laws in the first place.

A few years ago, we hung a giant sign in front of our Austin clinic that read, "Good women have abortions." This sign created more of a ripple effect in the pro-choice community than among antiabortion activists. Other providers, pro-choice activists, and Democrats were stunned when we put up this sign—stunned that we would be "so bold." But we are not ashamed; abortion should not be a secret. Good women do have abortions every day—and we providers are right here with them. We do not step away from the conflicts, challenges, or messy stuff. In fact, we see firsthand every day how transformational good abortion care can be for people. Through a framework of compassion and support, we deliver women into their futures.

Notes

1. In Alabama, Arizona, Arkansas, Indiana, Kansas, Kentucky, Louisiana, Michigan, Mississippi, Missouri, North Carolina, Ohio, Oklahoma, Pennsylvania, Rhode Island, South Carolina, South Dakota, Tennessee, Texas, and Utah, state legislators passed laws requiring that abortion clinics meet ASC standards. "Targeted Regulation of Abortion Providers" (New York: Guttmacher Institute, 2020), https://www.guttmacher.org/state-policy/explore/targeted-regulation-abortion-providers#.
2. Dan Grossman, K. White, K. Hopkins, and J. Potter, "The Public Health Threat of Anti-abortion Legislation," *Contraception* 89, no. 2 (2014): 73–74; Dan Grossman, S. Baum, L. Fuentes, K. White, K., Hopkins, A. Stevenson, and J. Potter, "Change in Abortion Services after Implementation of a Restrictive Law in Texas," *Contraception* 90, no. 5 (2014): 496–501.
3. Whole Woman's Health v. Hellerstedt, 579 U.S. 582 (2016).
4. Lawrence Hurley, "Supreme Court Firmly Backs Abortion Rights, Tosses Texas Law," Reuters, June 28, 2016), https://www.reuters.com/article/us-usa-court-abortion-idUSKCN0ZC0JL.

Chapter 5

Improving Abortion Care One Clinic at a Time

Renee Chelian

My intention is to talk about my clinics not just surviving but remaining optimistic in the face of adversity. We not only share the "We are in it to win it" attitude, but we are creating an atmosphere in our clinics as though there is *no* adversity. We have intentionally created and are moving forward as "Incubators for Change." In our incubator we offer much to our patients, the medical community, and the community at large. We do so much more on a daily basis than provide abortion care.

For multiple reasons, these are horrific times for many of the country's abortion providers. It would be very easy to lose all hope and live in despair or just close our doors. Even if a clinic or state is not facing a huge obstacle at the moment, we live in fear of the *next* bad piece of legislation, the *next* election, or the *next* court decision. In my three clinics, even when we are at our most optimistic, we are often in a state of posttraumatic stress disorder over recent TRAP [targeted regulation of abortion providers] laws and have had many discussions about "practicing to the law" instead of "to the patient." We also live in fear of the next inspection.

Of course, there are bright spots for us: the attorneys who defend us, the women we care for and their families, the allies and other advocates in my own state, and more recently the professional allies for independent providers, who have come to understand who we are, the value of our work, and our place in this profession. All of these people are among the reasons we hang on and find hope.

One of the physicians I work with was interviewed along with five other women physicians for an online piece called "5 Women Physicians Explain

Why They Became Abortion Providers."[1] She was pretty much the only one who explained that she came into this work very serendipitously, no profound reasons or experiences. In the last paragraph of her short interview she added,

> I feel saddened that abortion care can't just be incorporated into a woman's regular physician care [like any other medical treatment]. I'm very happy with the way things are going now though. The environment you have to set up to continually ensure that the patient has both the best medical care and the best supportive care for her decision can be very daunting. At this point we do a good job of addressing those needs and it would be hard to replicate that in a private setting.

When the article came out, she shared with me an email she sent to the journalist. Her response, she felt, seemed too simple to her after reading what the other women physicians reported as their reasons for becoming providers. And so she wrote a well-thought-out statement comparing "regular medicine" and "abortion medicine" with examples. It was smart, and it was wise. But, personally, I think it would be impossible to provide the kind of abortion care we do in a private doctor's office. And frankly I have never wanted to see abortion as part of everyday medicine because I believe that *it is* a specialty requiring special knowledge, experience, caring support staff, and other components that doctor' offices would find hard to offer, especially to large numbers of women.

I recognize that the "antis" have spent forty years shaming women and leading many to feel stigma. Maybe that would be different if every doctor did abortions as part of their practice. But if abortions were offered in every doctor's office, I doubt that we would have seen D&E [dilation and evacuation] practices move limits of gestation up and develop new protocols to improve safety and patient satisfaction. I doubt that continuing studies for off-label use of medication abortion and increased gestational limits would have happened. I cannot imagine a doctor's office helping to raise funds for low-income women whose lives are very messy and who show up more weeks pregnant and with less money than they scheduled for. These things, among others, have happened because we provide abortion as a specialty care and we continually challenge ourselves to be better and safer at our work and we do an unbelievable amount of care that could be considered "social services."

I love that our doctor's interview does not have an abortion story or some life-altering experience that made her want to become an abortion provider. None of the five doctors I work with do abortions because of some life-shaping moment. They do them because women need them, because it is the right thing to do, and because abortion is the specialty they chose to practice.

When I opened the first Northland Clinic in 1976, my vision was to make the world a better place for women. Over the years, we have added many ways to accomplish our vision and mission. But in the last year, we intentionally expanded and broadened our vision because we know that we are the best ones to fill the needs of the women and of the community. We have not closed ourselves to new ideas, and we do not shy away from opportunities to do and to help and to reach for more. Our perspective is that as true agents of change we not only make our clinical care better, but we affect the larger more long-term goals of our profession. The last difficult years have crystalized this for us.

Our doctors were ready for something more than day-to-day struggling, and I was ready to use my leadership skills for a new vision. As an independent provider, we can dream and brainstorm and make changes happen fast. It all came together at a time we felt was right and so we nurtured our dreams and went from a place of survival to becoming an Incubator for Change!

Our incubator image reminds us to remain positive because in our daily work we impact the world. We feel pride in our good patient care and still remain open to new ways to make it better. It excites us to have the opportunity to educate and teach not only our trainees but our advocate partners and the public at large. And our incubator image feels proactive. Our Incubator for Change includes the following:

1. First and foremost, we are always providing the best and most up-to-date abortion care. This includes the kind of counseling we can all be proud of. I only have to read the comments from patients that we post on our Facebook page to remind myself we are meeting this goal daily.

2. We are training and teaching. This helps to nurture the soul of our physicians and is important to them personally. We all feel a tremendous responsibility not only to mentor and teach the next generation but to dispel the myths and stigma that residents and medical students often have. We give them an opportunity to know who we are, who our patients are, and why we do what we do. We don't just teach them how to empty a uterus. They learn that there is so much more to our work. It is not only teaching residents and medical students; our nursing director also is interested in starting a chapter of Nursing Students for Choice, and we will support her efforts.

3. We do medical research, and we love the social science research we have participated in.

4. Advocacy work is central to our incubator. More than thirty years of experience working in advocacy have given me a lot of credibility

and working knowledge, but it was usually just me. For a long time, our physicians did not understand the impact they could and should have. Now, three of our current physicians have completed the Reproductive Health Leadership training and are becoming vocal advocates for abortion care and rights. They want to have a voice and are grateful for the support of each other and the support of the clinic and staff. One of them works closely with American College of Obstetricians and Gynecologists (ACOG), and all of them have helped create an atmosphere where speaking out feels safe for them.

We have been instrumental in starting and funding a new women's coalition, Michigan Lead. Michigan Lead has been bringing together a large number of groups to work together to advance issues that concern women and not let abortion be the divisive issue it has been in the past. There is much potential there. My daughter was hired as the codirector of this coalition, and she brings experience from the patient and provider world that has been lacking in leadership with these coalitions in the past. She also brings the voice of independent providers and is the fastest contact to our physicians when their voices are needed.

5. We recently started a Long Action Reversible Contraception (LARC) program through Reproductive Health Education in Family Medicine (RHEDI). This program is meaningful to our physicians, especially those who are former fellows.

6. Since late 2012, we have partnered with a private pro-choice adoption agency and we have placed more than twenty-five babies from our clinics. This program is meaningful to our counseling staff as they have real options for our patients who are too far in the pregnancy for an abortion and will now not be subjected to shame if adoption is an option they would like to consider. We are working with a documentary filmmaker who is interested in the idea that an abortion provider really does care about the woman's choice, no matter which choice, as long as it is her own.

7. We will continue to grow our gynecology clinic and offer new and needed services, and our new clinician is excited to have real input into women's health care.

I don't know what our future will hold. I won't bury my head in the sand, but I also will not let fear keep us from moving forward. From experience, I know that Northland will work with our allies to make proposed legislation better or fight back to stop the legislation. Or if a challenge is possible, we will challenge it with the Center for Reproductive Rights. Or we will find ways to comply and continue to offer the best abortion care in a supportive atmosphere for our patients, our staff, and our doctors.

In addition, Northland finances all these programs with income from patient fees. Abortion services are definitely our economic tool to cover the cost of our incubator activities. Of course, this leads to concerns about how the next piece of legislation affects our income and patient numbers and the money to cover these valuable goals. For now, I make it work.

Our incubator image has made us all happier. It helps balance the anti-stuff we deal with daily. We feel excited and recharged because we spend our time and energy on the goals we set. We still have to comply with the "regulatory stuff," but it is no longer the thing that we dwell on. We deal with it and go back to the incubator goals, which feed our souls. We are a much happier and stronger team.

In the big picture to continue our Incubator for Change, it was crucial that I have a succession plan—people who will ensure the continued success of the work and the vision I started and that we have all re-created—in the event of the unexpected. I have a responsibility to the women in my state. I have a responsibility to all the people who have supported me all these years, to my staff, and our physicians, all of whom are working to take back women's reproductive health care "One Clinic at a Time."

Note

1. Robin Marty, "5 Women Physicians Explain Why They Became Abortion Providers," *Cosmopolitan*, March 10, 2015, https://www.cosmopolitan.com/politics/news /a37549/why-these-five-women-became-abortion-providers/.

Part 3

Conscience

In June 1973, five months after the *Roe v. Wade* decision, President Nixon signed the Health Programs Extension Act into law. The act, which extended funding of a dozen public health programs, contained the so-called Church Amendment prohibiting discrimination against health care workers who refuse to provide abortion care on the basis of their moral convictions.[1] Since the passage of the Church Amendment, we have equated conscience in abortion and reproductive health care services with health care professionals' refusal to provide these services. As Sara Dubow's essay in this section illustrates, passage of the Church Amendment was not without controversy, and supporters of abortion voted for it at a time when abortion was far less controversial and political than it is today. But as the essays in this section will also illustrate, abortion providers, too, argue that their conscience influences their work—their conscience tells them to provide abortion care.

Conscience has long played a role in abortion care. In the late 1960s, a group of clergy came together to form the Clergy Consultation Service (CCS), an underground referral service made up of clergy from a wide range of denominations spread across the country: liberal Protestant ministers, Jewish rabbis, and dissident Catholic nuns and priests. Founded in 1967 by Reverend Howard Moody, an American Baptist senior pastor of Judson Memorial Church in New York City, CCS members were driven by their conscience to help women obtain illegal abortions prior to *Roe*. Women seeking illegal abortions could approach clergy affiliated with CCS to receive counseling and a referral to a safe abortion provider in the United States or abroad. By the time the U.S. Supreme Court decriminalized abortion, CCS had helped between 250,000 and 500,000 women receive safe abortions.[2]

Because clergy and abortion providers working with CCS were breaking the law, they clearly articulated their moral framework in defense of abortion. Grounded in situational ethics, clergy and physicians argued that women with unwanted pregnancies merited concern and help. To force them to carry an unwanted pregnancy to term constituted a "huge injustice." The most caring action, they held, was to support women's choice of abortion by helping them find an abortion provider. As the essay by Curtis Boyd and Glenna Halvorson-Boyd illustrates, prior to the legalization of abortion some abortion providers offered abortion services in secret. The pervasiveness of sex discrimination and the fact that women carried the burden of unwanted pregnancy meant that women regularly found their educational and career opportunities forestalled, felt overburdened with the care of children, or were locked into abusive relationships as a result of pregnancy and childbearing. Some physicians, like Curtis Boyd, secretly performed illegal abortions because they found that women operated at a disadvantage compared with men. "It wasn't a fair world for women," Curtis Boyd explains. "Her life is radically and drastically changed [as a result of pregnancy], which didn't apply to the man."[3]

The legalization of abortion led to a shift in emphasis. Supporters of legal abortion began to focus their arguments on rights and privacy—as articulated by the Supreme Court decision—while the antiabortion movement took up arguments emphasizing morality. To highlight the gruesome nature of abortion and the humanity of the fetus, antiabortion activists created a storyline that recounted the abortion experience from the perspective of the fetus. Even before the spread of ultrasound technology led to the proliferation of fetal imagery, fictional accounts invited readers to identify with the fetus, thus creating narratives that seemed to make visible what a lack of images rendered otherwise invisible. These accounts read consciousness of the abortion event into the fetal mind, insinuating, for instance, that the fetus understood the full danger of a needle or suction tip appearing in the uterus and would fight against it with all its might. While in some accounts the fetus struggled against medical instruments, in others it imagined a beautiful life on earth, only to experience the abortion as a betrayal by its mother.[4]

With the rise of ultrasound in the 1980s, antiabortion activists could also draw on visuals to illustrate their narration of abortion from the fetal perspective. Although ultrasound was developed as a medical diagnostic technology, ultrasound images of the fetus quickly acquired broader cultural meaning. Antiabortion activists expected that the ultrasound image had the power to transform the viewer. Indeed, the idea that knowledge of fetal life and the confrontation with the visual image would convert a woman to a prolife position has been central in right-to-life tactics.[5]

As the use of ultrasound exploded in the 1980s, antiabortion activists turned to the increasingly sophisticated technique to provide the public with a view of abortion from the perspective of the fetus. The 1984 antiabortion movie *The Silent Scream*, for instance, offered viewers supposedly real-time ultrasound images of a first-trimester abortion. Former abortion provider and now antiabortion narrator Bernard Nathanson focused the viewer's attention on a grainy freeze-frame, impossible to identify by the untrained eye, explaining that the image showed "the silent scream of a child threatened imminently with extinction."[6] Here, too, the fiction of fetal consciousness and idea that a fetus can experience a sense of betrayal were central to the narrative.

If antiabortion activists accorded fetuses in these narratives the same value as infants, they described women who had abortions as naïve and in need of protection. Indeed, they characterized women as incapable of making the decision to end a pregnancy. In the early 1980s, Nancyjo Mann, a singer in the Christian hard rock band Barnabas, founded the organization Women Exploited by Abortion (WEBA) to give voice to women who regretted their abortions. Mann herself had had an abortion in 1974 at the age of twenty-one. She had been pregnant with her third child, and her second husband had just walked out on her. Mann had wanted to keep the pregnancy but had followed the advice of her mother who, worried about her daughter's ability to support herself and her two children with no more than a high school degree, had urged Mann to end her third pregnancy. Mann, at that point five-and-a-half months pregnant, describes herself as traumatized by the abortion. Concluding that she had murdered her child, her life spiraled downward; she began to deal drugs, burglarized houses, and turned to prostitution. Only after finding God, Mann maintained, was she able to regain control of her life.[7] WEBA was made up solely of women who, like Mann, had had abortions and regretted them. Members were encouraged to speak publicly about their experiences and find reconciliation and healing through their engagement in the antiabortion movement.

In the mid-1980s, psychologist David C. Reardon conducted a survey of 252 WEBA members and published his research results in his 1987 book *Aborted Women: Silent No More*. Reardon constructed a story of women's abortion experiences that simultaneously presented the women as passive victims of abortion—and hence not responsible for their own actions—while also asserting that abortion was the killing of children and that these women were murderers. Because they were victims of abortion, WEBA members were not responsible for their abortions, nor for any criminal activity or child neglect they committed as a result of their postabortion trauma. Being a passive victim represented the only acceptable role women could play in relation to abortion and its aftermath. Most WEBA members alleged that they had not themselves chosen abortion but had been pressured by boyfriends, husbands, abortion counselors, or others to have an abortion. Indeed, to emphasize their passivity, Reardon referred to WEBA members as "the aborted." This stood in sharp contrast to his characterization of women who did not regret their abortions as "aborters," emphasizing their active participation in the process.[8] Once at the abortion clinic, women contended that they did not realize the procedure was killing a fetus until their confrontation with the dead body. Since antiabortion activists claimed that women would never choose abortion if they understood the outcome of the procedure, it was important to depict women as so naïve and innocent that they failed to recognize that abortion resulted in the death of the fetus. Women emerged from the experience feeling deceived, filled with guilt, and suffering physically and psychologically for years to come.[9]

The women described in Reardon's book are striking in their inability to take responsibility and choose for themselves. Indeed, *Aborted Women* paints portraits of women who are either so needy and dependent as to be paralyzed in their decision making or who, having chosen to have an abortion against the counsel of husbands or parents, were ready to blame others, usually the abortion provider or counselor, for making the wrong choice. What the portraits have in common is the suggestion that women were, indeed, unable to make the abortion decision.

Notwithstanding the accusation by abortion opponents that abortion providers acted immorally and unethically, ethical issues remained central to abortion providers after the legalization of abortion. Ethical issues emerged most firmly as abortion providers developed and debated abortion procedures after the first trimester. The more developed the fetus, the more likely abortion providers were to grapple with the ethical implications of their work. At the 1983 annual National Abortion Federation (NAF) meeting the issue of moral and ethical dilemmas of abortion stood front and center. "We believe it serves us well to ponder complex moral issues, to sharpen our sense of moral rightness and to become aware of how our personal moral limits affect our interactions with patients," NAF's executive director noted as she introduced the first panel.[10] The panelists suggested ways to think about the concept of personhood. Personhood, Marjorie Reilly Maguire, PhD, a fellow in ethics and theology at Catholics for a Free Choice, suggested, should be thought of in relational terms. She argued that a fetus becomes a person "at the moment when the mother gives consent to the pregnancy. Before this point what you have is a purely biological development going on within her body."[11] Developmental biologist Clifford Grobstein noted that the concept of person was only partly biological, and even the biological components came gradually into existence. "Forceful and integrated behavior," he told the NAF audience, "such as we associate with persons in the usual context, seems first to appear mid-way in the third trimester—along with maturational changes in the upper brain."[12]

Because dilation and evacuation (D&E) procedures, by 1980 the most common second-trimester abortion procedure, involved the extraction of recognizable fetal parts, the procedure took an emotional toll on the doctors, as a study of the emotional impact of D&Es pointed out:

> A physician performing a D&E must deal with the second trimester fetus in an intimate, physical way, using methods of evacuation that often take longer than amniocentesis and that may be distasteful to the medical staff. Ossified parts, such as the skull, must often be crushed. The bone fragments must be extracted carefully to avoid tearing the cervix. Reconstruction of the fetal sections after removal from the uterus is necessary to ensure completeness of the abortion procedure."[13]

Some abortion providers had no problems performing D&Es. Others felt comfortable performing first-trimester vacuum aspirations but uncomfortable performing a D&E because it entailed the process of dismembering a fetus.

NAF addressed the issue of the emotional burdens of D&E head on. Its seminars on D&E services included workshops on ethical considerations, operative technique, the use of laminaria, the development of standards for D&E services, and counseling and staff training. At a 1984 risk seminar on D&E, the faculty gave advice on how to prepare staff for the performance of D&Es, how to facilitate staff acceptance of second trimester abortions, how to present second trimester abortions to patients, and how to help staff voice their feelings, identify emotional barriers, and select coping techniques to handle the stress of providing D&E services. Such a broad approach meant that physicians and clinic staff not only gained valuable skills but also received important emotional support.

Abortion providers and their supporters also recognized that women's decisions to end a pregnancy were moral decisions. At a 1985 NAF meeting, feminist theologian Carter Heyward contended that good theology and good morality was rooted in lived experience and in a consideration of the effects of our decisions and actions.[14] Feminist theologian and academic Virginia Ramey Mollenkott pleaded that women's moral agency deserved respect: "To deny decision-making to a pregnant woman is to disrespect the integrity of her conscience and ultimately to deny her full personhood." Mollenkott explained,

> Pregnant women are faced with deciding whether or not they can maintain a covenant of caring with the fetus they have conceived. Since a newborn infant needs not only physical care but also psychological attention and tender affect, and since the covenant with a child is life-long, only the woman involved is capable of determining the probability of living up to that covenant—or should she give the baby up for adoption, whether or not she can endure the life-long anxiety about her child's welfare.[15]

Women, these speakers asserted, made careful and deliberate decisions about their own future and the future of the fetus they were carrying. They understood their moral obligation to be toward the fetus, and they chose to end pregnancies because they felt that it was the most ethical choice.

Women who sought abortions before and after *Roe* had significant reasons to do so. As the essay by Curtis Boyd and Glenna Halvorson-Boyd illustrates, women made a range of arguments for choosing abortion within the larger context of their lives and their responsibilities to other family members. Many felt that childbearing and child raising should take place in a familial context. "I decided to have an abortion because I had no relationship with the father and believed that having a child at that point in my life would have ruined the rest of it," one young woman argued.[16] Most had high expectations of themselves as mothers and sought an abortion because the realities of their lives meant that they were unable to meet their own expectations regarding parenthood. One woman in her mid-twenties, who initially had rejected her partner's desire for an abortion and planned to raise the child on her own, eventually changed her mind when the realities of single parenthood sunk in. "I decided to go through with the pregnancy and even started picking out names for my baby," she wrote in a notebook for patients laid out in the recovery room of a clinic. "At night though, I was feeling depressed and alone and began to realize the reality of wanting to raise a healthy baby in a supportive wholesome environment. I deserve to have a partner who loves me and wants to raise a baby with me. I deserve to continue my goals of becoming financially successful. I know that I will be a wonderful mother some day when I'm ready to prepare and plan."[17] Even women who had loving and supportive partners frequently felt that an unplanned pregnancy was not the right foundation for marriage and childbearing.[18]

A number of women seeking abortions tried to protect their children from abusive relationships or to escape such relationships altogether. "I knew this guy since high school," one mother of two explained her decision to have an abortion.

> He was my best friend until we took our relationship further. I became pregnant. My first [pregnancy] was complicated. He had changed. We would fight and I'd be blocked or shoved into walls. How I didn't lose my daughter is a mystery. When I had my last daughter, things turned for the worse. I was forced to have sex. If I said no, it would be a fight and forced sex. When I found out I was pregnant, I wanted to be happy. But I felt rage and hate. After I felt sad and alone. My parents aren't supportive. Thankfully my sister was. Being she was forced into rape [*sic*]. I won't lie, I still feel like shit. But I know this was for the best. I will miss my daughter, but I know she will be safe.[19]

Even if husbands were not abusive, many were unsupportive and of no help with family responsibilities and child raising. Women described husbands who were unreliable, drank, or were generally unhelpful, leaving women unwilling to take on the responsibilities for an additional child.[20] For many, becoming pregnant heightened their sense that they wanted to protect their future babies from a life of hardship. "I had always been against abortions but the feeling of pregnancy and being a mom gives you a sense of protection," one seventeen-year-old explained. "I feel in my situation I'm protecting my baby's life from a struggling household full of drama and speculation. I think of it as my baby being with God makes me so happy and relieved that my love is in heaven being take care of."[21]

Many women argued that their responsibilities to other family members—most often already existing children—precluded having more children. Some were the sole breadwinners for their families. "A new baby would have made all of us financially dependent whereas we were now independent," explained a mother of two who had just separated from her husband and was trying to negotiate single motherhood. "I felt it was important to be able to do well for 2 children rather than not much for 3. . . . It was best for my peace of mind. It meant my 2 children would have a life of quality rather than a mother with too many responsibilities. . . . They are lacking nothing, are very happy and well adjusted."[22]

But women did not merely seek to stay off welfare; they also sought to improve their education and get established in their career before devoting time to children. "I was four years into a career and had aspirations of returning to school full-time to receive an advanced degree," explained a twenty-nine-year-old mother who had two abortions. "Now that my child was 8 years old, I was relatively free to do this. I feel very strongly that an infant should have a parent at home at least half the time the first three years. My husband wants more children but is only willing to step out of his professional education for one year. I do not want any more children. I feel that my personal development is critical to our existing family unit. I would be very resentful of any unwanted children."[23]

Especially young women were also concerned about the impact a child outside marriage would have on parents and other family members. "Bearing this child unmarried," one young woman explained, "would have hurt and possibly ruined quite a few people's lives and possibly my father's good reputation, as he is well known and holds important positions in our state."[24]

Finally, women argued that they had a moral obligation to the children they were going to put into this world. Parents seeking to end wanted pregnancies after their fetus had been diagnosed with abnormalities saw their decision as protecting the fetus from unnecessary suffering. "We found out he had a severe heart defect that meant he would die slowly within a few days or weeks of being born," the husband of one patient wrote. "We couldn't bear the thought of watching a baby slowly suffocate and die just so we could see him and hold him. That would be selfish. We chose to terminate so that he would die painlessly inside his mother where he wouldn't ever know pain or suffering."[25] "If you know that this child will suffer more on earth than you will by having an abortion," one woman concluded, "then that is a decision for you to make and only you to make."[26]

Unable to provide their future children with the life they wanted, women framed their abortion decisions as a moral choice. "I felt that I did not want to bear a child without a father," one young woman explained. "I did not love the father, did not want to marry him, and, as a matter of fact, never even told him that I was pregnant. . . . I did not feel my abortion was immoral. . . . On the contrary, I felt it would be immoral to bring a child into the world under my circumstances."[27] Another young woman, who had a legal abortion at age fourteen, noted that she ended the pregnancy out of love for the fetus: "I was in love with the guy. He was 16. He loved me too, but we were too young to have a baby. . . . Marriage was out of the question. We were too young, he was black and I was white, we didn't have money. But we loved each other and that baby—that's why we didn't have it. It wouldn't have been fair to the baby."[28]

Women also worried about the feelings of their potential children should they decide to go through with pregnancy and childbearing and give the child up for adoption. "There are too many crazy people in the world and too many who already feel unwanted," one young woman noted. "An adopted person must have feelings of not being wanted and if a person can't raise their own child because they didn't want it in the first place, then they shouldn't have brought it into this world."[29]

The essay by Lisa Harris describes the impact that the stigmatization of abortion has on providers' ability to discuss their work. Physicians and staff who talk about the complications of and their feelings toward abortion found their words exploited by antiabortion activists such as Joseph Scheidler. Scheidler regularly attended NAF meetings, which until the late 1980s were open to anyone. There he closely followed the presentations of abortion providers and turned their words against them whenever possible. When abortion provider Warren Hern observed in a 1980 article about D&E, for instance, that "there is no possibility of denying an act of destruction," Scheidler repeated Hern's words as proof that abortion providers knew that abortion was murder.[30] Providers, who at times were disconcerted by the procedures they performed but were committed to a pro-choice position, had no space to voice their thoughts without the risk that such discussion would be exploited by the antiabortion movement. As a result, they grew silent.

As the essays by Shelley Sella and Lisa Harris illustrate, abortion providers understood their primary obligation to be toward the pregnant woman. They accorded respect to the fetus. At the same time, women and abortion providers could choose abortions despite conflicted feelings about the fetus. They felt that a woman's need to end an unwanted pregnancy outweighed considerations for the fetus. Many felt that later abortions were more serious than early abortions and hence required a defense. But those providers who offered abortions later in pregnancy also felt that declining a woman's request for abortion was, as Lisa Harris explains, "an act of unspeakable violence."[31]

Providers understood their own and women's decisions as moral decisions. The essays in this section speak to the ways in which providers' conscience helped them to do this work. As Lisa Harris notes, "While I was over and over accused of having no conscience, I realized that my crisis of conscience would come if I didn't do abortion work, if I abandoned women who needed care. In other words, I was a 'conscientious provider.'"

Notes

1. Health Programs Extension Act of 1973; Public Health Service Act Extension, Public Law 93–94, 93rd Congress, S. 1136.
2. Gillian Frank, *Making Choice Sacred: Liberal Religion and Reproductive Rights Before Roe v. Wade* (Chapel Hill: University of North Carolina Press, forthcoming); Carole Joffe, *Doctors of Conscience: The Struggle to Provide Abortion before and after Roe v. Wade* (Boston: Beacon Press, 1995); D. P. Cline, *Creating Choice: A Community Responds to the Need for Abortion and Birth Control, 1961–1973* (New York: Palgrave Macmillan, 2006).

3. Joffe, *Doctors of Conscience*, 89.

4. Johanna Schoen, *Abortion after Roe* (Chapel Hill: University of North Carolina Press, 2015), 140–144.

5. Faye D. Ginsburg, *Contested Lives: The Abortion Debate in an American Community* (Berkeley: University of California Press, 1989), 104.

6. Jack Duane Dabner, dir., *The Silent Scream* (Crusade for Life/American Portrait Films, 1984), available at https://www.youtube.com/watch?v=gON-8PP6zgQ.

7. David C. Reardon, *Aborted Women: Silent No More* (Wheaton, IL: Crossway Books, 1987), xxiii.

8. Reardon, *Aborted Women*, 68, 254. Reardon argued that women who were "completely satisfied" with their abortions are few and far between and that their claims must be taken with a grain of salt since to admit otherwise was to open the door to reevaluation, doubt, self-reproach, and despair. Some women, he held, suffered from their abortions on a subconscious level and were "walking time-bombs" waiting to explode over situations seemingly unrelated to their previous abortion. Women least likely to suffer from abortion, he concluded, were women who showed little motherliness and were aggressive rather than nurturing. They were likely to be self-centered and property oriented, rather than people oriented, and extremely manipulative of others. They suffered least not because they were more psychologically stable but because they were already so psychologically crippled (*Aborted Women*, 118–119, 138–139).

9. Reardon, *Aborted Women*.

10. National Abortion Federation (NAF) Quarterly, Summer 1983, file NAF 1983, series Abortion, Takey Crist Papers, Sally Bingham Center for Women's History and Culture, Duke University Libraries, Durham, NC.

11. NAF Quarterly, Summer 1983.

12. NAF Quarterly, Summer 1983.

13. Judith Bourne Rooks and Willard Cates Jr., "3. Emotional Impact if D&Es vs. Instillation," *Family Planning Perspectives* 9, no. 6 (1977): 276–277, https://doi.org/10.2307/2134349.

14. C. Heyward, "Abortion: A Moral Choice," in National Abortion Federation 9th Annual Meeting, 10 June 1985, Boston, MA. Box: Speeches and Resources, Terry Beresford Papers, Sally Bingham Center for Women's History and Culture, Duke University Libraries, Durham, NC.

15. Virginia Ramey Mollenkott, "Respecting the Moral Agency of Women," Religious Coalition for Abortion Rights Educational Fund Inc., 1987. Box 93, Folder 4, NARAL Papers, Schlesinger Library, Cambridge, MA.

16. Rose Soma, *Women Speak Out about Abortion: By Women, for Women in their Own Words*, ([Miller Place, NY: R. Soma], 1978), 17, and also see 19, 31. Rose Soma, a writer and journalist, collected letters from women reflecting on their reasons for ending a pregnancy in the late 1970s, as legislators debated passage of a Human Life Amendment hoping to overturn the *Roe v. Wade* decision.

17. 2010 Purple Notebook, 65, Mountain County Women's Clinic, Susan Wicklund Papers, Sally Bingham Center for Women's History and Culture, Duke University Libraries, Durham, NC.

18. Soma, *Women Speak Out*, 59.

19. 2013 Brown Notebook, 20; see also: 2016 Red Notebook, both: Southwest Women's Option [in author's possession], 4.

20. Soma, *Women Speak Out*, 11, 83, 6. See also Johanna Schoen, "Abortion Care as Moral Work," *Journal of Modern European History* 17, no. 3 (2019): 262–279, https://doi.org/10.1177/1611894419854304.

21. 2010 Yellow Notebook, Southwest Women's Option [in author's possession], 15–16.

22. Soma, *Women Speak Out*, 22; also see pp. 17, 25 (for a widow with one child who had six illegal abortions, most of them in her twenties, to stay off welfare), 58, 62.

23. Soma, *Women Speak Out*, 39; also see 37.

24. Soma, *Women Speak Out*, 40.

25. 2015 Brown Notebook 3, Southwest Women's Option [in author's possession], 10.

26. 2015 Brown Notebook 3, Southwest Women's Option [in author's possession], 5.

27. Soma, *Women Speak Out*, 48.

28. Soma, *Women Speak Out*, 47.

29. Soma, *Women Speak Out*, 9.

30. Warren M. Hern and B. Corrigan, "What about Us? Staff Reactions to D&E," *Advances in Planned Parenthood* 15, no. 1 (1980): 3–8, here 7; Joe Scheidler's presentation, Atlanta, GA, January 12, 1986, Stone Mountain Community Church, Folder: Joseph Scheidler, Susan Hill Papers, Sally Bingham Center for Women's History and Culture, Duke University Libraries, Durham, NC.

31. Lisa H. Harris, "Second Trimester Abortion Provision: Breaking the Silence and Changing the Discourse," supplement, *Reproductive Health Matters* 16, no. 31 (2008): 74–81, https://doi.org/10.1016/s0968-8080(08)31396-2, here 78.

Chapter 6

From Conscience Clauses to Conscience Wars

Sara Dubow

Championing the rights of those demanding exemptions from laws that conflict with their religious beliefs was a key promise of Donald Trump's presidential campaign in 2016 and has been a central project of the Trump administration.[1] In the context of reproductive health care, that project has involved expanding the exemptions to the Affordable Care Act's contraceptive mandate and enforcing protections for health care providers who have religious objections to participating in abortion care. On May 4, 2017, President Trump called upon the Secretary of Health and Human Services (HHS) to "consider issuing amended regulations, consistent with applicable law, to address conscience-based objections to the preventive-care mandate" of the Affordable Care Act.[2] On May 2, 2019, the HHS Office for Civil Rights (OCR) issued a rule that, in their words, "protects individuals and health care entities from discrimination on the basis of their exercise of conscience in HHS-funded programs," and "implements full and robust enforcement of approximately 25 provisions passed by Congress protecting longstanding conscience rights in healthcare."[3] OCR Director Roger Severino, who had previously served as the Director of the DeVos Center for Religion and Civil Society at the Heritage Foundation, heralded the new rules this way: "Finally, laws prohibiting government funded discrimination against conscience and religious freedom will be enforced like every other civil rights law. This rule ensures that health care entities and professionals won't be bullied out of the health care field because they decline to participate in actions that violate their conscience, including the taking of human life."[4]

    The Trump administration matched this heightened rhetorical commitment to protecting those health care providers with a dramatic increase of

administrative resources. On January 18, 2018, HHS announced the establishment of a new Conscience and Religious Freedom Division (CRFD) under the
OCR.[5] Between 2008 and 2016, the OCR received a total of ten complaints
related to conscience and religious freedom provisions; between 2016 and
2018, the office received thirty-four complaints. According to the 2020 Fiscal
Report, the newly established CFRD received 343 complaints of conscience
violations and 441 complaints involving religious freedom and religious discrimination in its first year, an increase that reflected the new outreach and
enforcement priorities of the new office.[6] In fiscal year 2018, in its first year
the CRFD had been allocated $602,000; in fiscal year 2019, its budget was
$2.148 million, an increase of 256 percent. The fiscal year 2020 budget request
is $4.8 million. The CRFD staff has grown from one person in 2018 to six
people in 2019 to twelve people in 2020.[7]

One of the first complaints investigated by this new office involved a law
that has been on the books since 1973: the Church Amendment to the Public
Health Service Act, which prevented hospitals receiving federal funds or individuals working in those hospitals from being forced to provide or participate
in abortion or sterilization procedures if doing so would be contrary to their religious beliefs or moral convictions.[8] On May 9, 2018, on behalf of an unnamed
Catholic nurse, the American Center for Law and Justice (ACLJ, an organization
whose chief counsel was Jay Sekulow, President Trump's personal lawyer) filed
with the OCR a "Complaint for Discrimination in Violation of 42 U.S.C § 300a-
7(c)(1) ('Church Amendment')."[9] According to the complaint, despite the fact
that the nurse had previously told her employer, the University of Vermont Medical Center (UVMMC), that she could not participate in abortion procedures
because of her religious beliefs, she "had been coerced by her employer, University of Vermont Medical Center, Inc., into participating in an abortion." Alleg-
ing that she feared being charged with patient abandonment and losing her job
and license, the complaint explains that the nurse "participated under duress . . .
suffered immediate emotional distress, attempted to suppress the event psychologically, and has been haunted by nightmares ever since."[10]

In August 2019, the HHS OCR issued a Notice of Violation letter finding
that the UVMMC had in fact violated the Church Amendment in this case.[11] Jay
Sekulow praised the finding: "HHS's Office of Civil Rights has, at long last, put
teeth in a law [Church Amendment] that has lain largely dormant since its
enactment."[12] The hospital has challenged the finding, saying that the hospital
"has robust, formal protections that safeguard both our employees' religious,
ethical, and cultural beliefs, and our patients' rights to access safe and legal
abortion. . . . When the UVM Medical Center first learned of the allegation that

are the subject of the OCR's letter, we promptly and thoroughly investigated them and determined that they were not supported by the facts."[13] This particular case is not yet resolved, and it seems likely that it will be the first of many to come—either because the Church Amendment is in fact being violated with increasing frequency or because of the heightened outreach of the OCR.

This particular case offers an opportunity to revisit the "largely dormant" Church Amendment. From the vantage point of 2019, the highly politicized and almost completely partisan fights over the issue of conscientious objection and religious exemptions in the context of the provision of reproductive health care are entirely predictable. These fights, though, stand in stark contrast to the passage of and reactions to that first conscience clause, the Church Amendment, which was passed by a nearly unanimous and entirely bipartisan vote in the spring of 1973. In explaining how and why the conscience clause meant something different in 1973 than it does in 2019, I ask if, perhaps, the 1973 debate offers lessons for thinking about today's conscience wars.

On June 18, 1973, five months after the Supreme Court issued the *Roe v. Wade* decision, President Nixon signed into law the Health Programs Extension Act, which extended for one year the funding of a dozen public health programs. This act included for the first time a federal conscience clause that would allow health care providers and federally funded institutions to refuse to perform or provide abortions or sterilizations for reasons of religious belief or moral conviction.[14] The conscience clause had been added to the bill in an amendment proposed by Senator Frank Church, a Democrat from Idaho; it was debated by Congress throughout the spring of 1973. The Senate passed what has come to be known as the Church Amendment by a vote of 92:1. The House of Representatives passed it by a vote of 372:1.[15] Over the next year, Congress would attach a similar clause to the Foreign Assistance Act, the National Service Research Act, and the Legal Services Act. Over the next several years, almost every state would pass some version of a conscience clause.[16]

At the time, this first conscience clause received very little media attention.[17] But two years later, in a 1975 cover story focusing on the prolife movement's largely unsuccessful efforts to pass a Human Life Amendment, *Newsweek* magazine singled out this act, writing that "only a conscience clause measure sponsored by Idaho's Democratic Senator Frank Church has had far-reaching effect."[18] That far-reaching effect continues to be felt today. The huge literature—mostly by legal scholars and bioethicists—on conscience clauses in general and the contraceptive mandate in particular—is, for the most part, normative and prescriptive, and typically identifies the 1973 Church Amendment as significant primarily as a historical precedent.[19] By contrast, I will examine understanding the passage of the Church Amendment as a historical event on its own terms in its own moment.

At a moment when debates over conscience clauses have erupted into the highly politicized and almost completely partisan phenomenon that the Heritage Foundation has called "conscience wars," it seems worth thinking about how and why a conscience clause was passed nearly unanimously forty years ago.[20] Although it is true that this first conscience clause received nearly unanimous bipartisan support, it is also true that it generated intense debate and some significant opposition. Several legislators who ultimately voted for it raised serious concerns about its constitutionality and its potentially dangerous consequences for women's health and rights. Examining both the public unanimity and the behind-the-scenes opposition offers a new perspective on the forces shaping abortion politics in the immediate aftermath of *Roe v. Wade*, and, perhaps, a new way of thinking about the conflicts shaping our current political and legal landscape.

The legislative history of the Church Amendment offers a window into a moment in time when the Democratic-led Congress—focused on escalating confrontations with the Nixon administration over Watergate, Vietnam, the relationship between executive power and legislative authority, and the budget while fighting Nixon's efforts to build a new political majority—was also beginning to grapple with the intrusion of the abortion issue in national politics through the *Roe* decision. At that same time, Democrats and Republicans in Congress were passing an unprecedented number of laws banning sex discrimination and enacting a series of federal protections for women's rights, raising the complicated question of how legalized abortion would intersect with this legislative effort to define and ensure women's equality. These political forces shaped the legislative debate over the meaning of the necessity, constitutionality, and scope of the Church Amendment.

In 1973, it was not at all inevitable that the Democratic Party would become identified as the pro-choice party and the Republican Party would become identified as the prolife party. A 1972 Gallup poll found that 68 percent of Republicans and 59 percent of Democrats believed that abortion should be a decision between a woman and her physician.[21] In fact, Republicans had historically been more supportive of legalized abortion than Democrats. That was in the process of changing. In 1972, following the advice of his aides who wanted to lure northern Catholic voters to the Republican Party, Nixon reversed his earlier relaxation on an abortion ban in military facilities and joined the attacks on George McGovern as the radical candidate of "amnesty, abortion, and acid."[22]

But although the realignment of the parties on this issue was beginning to take shape, it was far from complete. And at this particular moment of flux, legislators on all sides of the abortion issue chose not to turn the vote on the conscience clause into a referendum on abortion in general, or *Roe* in particular. Framing their support for the Church Amendment not as a vote for or against legalized abortion but as a vote for religious freedom had strategic advantages for both parties and legislators.

Some key legislators expressed a degree of ambivalence about the *Roe v. Wade* decision and were eager to distance themselves from it. The conscience clause offered them a way to do that while making clear their support for religious freedom trumped their support for legalized abortion. As Church said, "nothing is more fundamental to our national birthright than freedom of religion." For example, Senator Adlai Stevenson III (D-Illinois) began his remarks supporting the conscience clause by expressing his personal opposition to "abortion on demand" after the first trimester, and criticizing the judicial overreach of the *Roe* decision. Legislators like Church and Stevenson, who at least in limited ways supported legalized abortion, wanted their support for the conscience clause to highlight the fact that their commitment to religious freedom transcended their support for legalized abortion. Republicans who opposed legalized abortion wanted their support for the conscience clause to be understood as an example of their willingness to find common ground. James Buckley (Conservative-New York), a leader of the prolife movement, went out of his way to avoid railing against *Roe* when he praised Church for sponsoring this "most important and timely" amendment.

For a brief moment in 1973, both prolife and pro-choice legislators saw the conscience clause as a way to diffuse rather than escalate abortion politics—as a way to find common ground rather than as a way to exaggerate political differences. This moment was very brief. The same day that the conscience clause was passed in the House of Representatives, Buckley sponsored for the first time a so-called Human Life Amendment that would have overturned *Roe* had it passed.

That moment was also not entirely consensual. How do we understand those individuals who opposed the conscience clause but ultimately voted for it? Several legislators had concerns. Bella Abzug, a Democrat from New York and a strong supporter of legalized abortion, spoke out against the conscience clause but ultimately voted for it. Examining why Abzug put aside her opposition illustrates the complicated way that women's rights activists responded to the *Roe* decision.[23]

Unlike today, in 1973 there was strong bipartisan support for legislation supporting women's rights.[24] In 1971, the House had approved the Equal Rights Amendment (ERA) by a bipartisan vote of 354 to 24 and the Senate approved it by a bipartisan vote of 84 to 8 in 1972.[25] Both the Republican and Democratic Party platforms of 1972 supported the ERA. In 1972 and 1973, Congress, with bipartisan support, had passed legislation prohibiting sex discrimination in federally funded job training programs, legislation that extended to domestic workers the minimum wage provisions of the Fair Labor Standards Act, and Title IX which prohibited sex discrimination in federally funded educational programs.[26]

Bella Abzug was one of the strongest advocates for these causes and also for the legalization of abortion. Her strong and frequent statements opposing the conscience clause make her ultimate vote for it quite surprising. In a letter to constituents who wrote to her about abortion, she wrote, "Clearly, no woman should be forced to have an abortion if her conscience forbids it, but no woman should be prevented from having an abortion because the conscience of some other individual would be offended by it."[27]

In the House debate, she made four arguments explaining why the conscience clause was unconstitutional. First, she argued that the conscience clause violated both "the rights of individual citizens to have abortions or sterilizations and the rights of physicians and other health care personnel to perform such procedures." She also argued that allowing federally funded hospitals to opt out of providing abortions was comparable to allowing federally funded hospitals to opt out of complying with civil rights laws, a practice which had been found to be unconstitutional in two recent district court cases.[28] She went on to make the case that the conscience clause privileged one set of religious beliefs over others, thus violating the establishment clause of the first amendment.[29] Finally, Abzug emphasized that this clause would "discriminate against persons of lesser means," arguing that "the clearest example of this is a woman who desires an abortion but whose local hospital—an institution receiving Federal funds—refuses to perform such operations. Unless she can afford to go to another hospital, perhaps hundreds of miles distant, her constitutional right will be rendered utterly meaningless."[30]

Abzug's objections were echoed by several women's rights organizations. The Women's Rights Project of the American Civil Liberties Union, the National Abortion Rights Action League, and Planned Parenthood all issued public statements opposing the conscience clause. The YWCA, the National Council for Jewish Women, the Religious Coalition for Abortion Rights, and Catholics for a Free Choice all wrote letters to Bella Abzug and other representatives articulating their support for abortion rights and opposition to the conscience clause.[31]

So it seems clear where Abzug and many of her organizational supporters stood on the issue. But she was also a co-sponsor of the Health Programs Extension Act. On the day of the House vote, she received a letter from Representative James Hastings, a Republican from New York, reminding her that "'freedom of conscience' language has been added to the bill . . . it is essential that it be passed."[32] Abzug was caught between her beliefs and political exigencies. I think that one reason Abzug might have decided to vote for the conscience clause is that she might have hoped that compromising on this issue might gain support for pending legislation on women's rights.

An exchange between Harriet Pilpel, an attorney with the ACLU Women's Rights Project, and Representative Robert Drinan, a Democrat from Massachusetts who was also a Jesuit priest, supports that possibility. Pilpel was opposed to the conscience clause and was writing a law review article criticizing its constitutionality.[33] Her files on the drafting of her article include a letter from Drinan, in which he explained that he thought the clause was "relatively harmless" and that provoking a floor fight on the issue would be ill advised because it might produce "adoption of disastrous language which could have catastrophic effects upon . . . the rights of women."[34]

Drinan's point was that a battle against the conscience clause would be inevitably lost and would have consequences for the larger struggle to advance women's rights. There was some hope that compromising on this issue might get some prolife legislators to support some of the other pending legislation on women's rights issues. Abzug's vote suggests that she agreed with Drinan that opposing the conscience clause might have too high a price.

Abzug was deeply invested in anti-gender-discrimination legislation that was pending on a wide range of issues, including access to credit and social security benefits.[35] Some of the women in Congress who were her allies in these efforts did not necessarily share her commitment to abortion rights in general or her opposition to the conscience clause in particular. There is a letter in her files from a woman who asked Abzug, "How do the other women in Congress stand on the abortion issue? . . . It would really be great if all of you would present a united front." At the bottom on that letter, Bella Abzug wrote, "Unfortunately not all the women members of Congress feel as I do about this issue."[36] Three of Abzug's greatest allies in the fight for a wide range of women's rights legislation, including the ERA, were Lindy Boggs (D-Louisiana), Margaret Heckler (R-Massachusetts), and Ella Grasso (D-Connecticut): all three opposed legalized abortion.

Abzug may have calculated that voting against the conscience clause that was going to pass with or without her vote was not worth the political capital she would expend. In the immediate context, that pragmatism may have made sense, but in the long term her concerns about the impact of the conscience clause on women's ability to access abortions were realized. In 2017, 89 percent of U.S. counties were without a clinic providing abortion care, and 38 percent of women between the ages of fifteen and forty-four lived in those counties.[37] For 2.5 million poor women, the nearest abortion provider is more than an hour away.[38] According to a 2014 study, 14.5 percent of all U.S. acute care hospitals are Catholic and follow the Ethical and Religious Directives for Catholic Health Services that prohibit abortions.[39]

A story about a woman from Manchester, New Hampshire, named Kathleen Prieskorn illustrates what these statistics mean under a particular set of circumstances. When she was three months pregnant, Prieskorn felt a trickle of fluid run down her leg. She rushed to the nearest hospital where her doctor determined that her amniotic sac had torn, triggering a miscarriage. He also detected a fetal heartbeat. Because the hospital had recently merged with a Catholic hospital and was obligated to comply with the Ethical and Religious Directives for Catholic Health Care Services, the doctor wasn't allowed to perform a uterine evacuation, despite the fact that the fetus had no possibility of surviving. The nearest hospital that would perform the procedure was eighty miles away. Prieskorn had no car and no health insurance, so the doctor gave her $400, and she took a cab. She describes the experience this way: "During that trip, which seemed endless, I was not only devastated, but terrified. I knew that if there were complications I could lose my uterus—and maybe even my life."[40] Prieskorn's experience is exactly what Bella Abzug had worried about when the first conscience clause was passed.

An aspect of this story worth examining is the role of the doctor who lent Kathleen Prieskorn the money. His willingness to do so suggests that he did not feel comfortable with the restraints placed on his conscience and his commitment to provide his patient with the best medical care. Senator Jacob Javits, a Republican of New York, who like Abzug opposed the conscience clause but ultimately voted for it, had anticipated this problem and had made some effort to ameliorate it. In the Senate debate, Javits spoke at great length about his concern that the conscience clause didn't protect physicians who wanted to provide abortions or sterilizations. He added a clause that would protect physicians who wanted to provide abortions at hospitals that allowed them to do so from losing their privileges at hospitals that didn't.[41] This nondiscrimination clause would not have allowed the doctor to perform the procedure that Prieskorn needed in this case, but it does suggest that even in 1973 there was an alternative way of conceptualizing acts of conscience.

Javits argued that there were doctors who believed that providing abortions was an act of conscience, and that restricting them from doing so impinged on their rights. One woman made a related argument in a letter she wrote to Abzug. "I am deeply distressed over the 'freedom of conscience' legislation," she wrote. "I consider it 'sinful' for a doctor or hospital to *refuse* to perform an abortion when a woman requests it. When tax money is given to support such a hospital or pay such a doctor, I become party, as a tax-payer, to such 'sin,' and I feel my conscience in this matter deserves as much consideration as that of the doctor or the hospital."[42]

So Javits approached the issue of conscience and abortion from the perspective of the physician, and the woman writing to Abzug approached it from the perspective of a taxpayer. Some abortion rights activists also thought about the conscience argument from the perspective of women seeking abortions. In 1972, Jimmey Kaye, the executive director of the Association for the Study of Abortion, wrote a memo discussing the "need to find a phrase to counter the Right to Life" slogan. Weighing the relative merits of two possibilities—the "Right to Choose" and "Freedom of Conscience"—Kaye argued that the "Right to Choose" was a better slogan for two reasons. "Right to Life is short, catchy, and is composed of monosyllabic words," she wrote. "We need something comparable. Right to Choose would seem to do the job." Her second reason was more complicated. "Conscience," she wrote, is "an internal matter while choice has to do with action—and it is action we are concerned with. A woman's conscience may well tell her abortion is wrong, but she may choose (and must have the right to choose) to have one anyway for compelling practical reasons. A woman's conscience may tell her that abortion is right, but she may choose to run the risk of having a . . . baby anyway."[43]

Abortion providers have increasingly begun to describe their work with the same language of conscience being invoked and deployed by those opposed to abortion.[44] One leading example is Dr. Willie Parker, a self-described Christian abortion provider, and one of the only providers in the deep south. Parker argues that providing abortions is an act of compassion, the conscientious provision of abortion requires the same level of protection as conscientious objection.[45] He writes, "It has not been easy watching the definition of conscience be oversimplified to mean refusal of vital health services for women on religious grounds. . . . The clarity I have about loving my neighbor as myself has been simply to want for women what I want for myself. I want a life of dignity, self-determination, well-being and the ability to participate in the common good. . . .

Providing abortion care when women request it is a primary way that I can preserve these possibilities. . . . My conscience demands it."[46] Dr. Lisa Harris
describes that abortion providers who, like herself, "have much to lose, facing
stigma, marginalization within medicine, harassment, and the threat of (or
actual) harm . . . continue to offer abortion care because deeply-held, core ethical beliefs compel them."[47] Nurse practitioner and abortion provider Monica
McLemore puts it this way: "I can attest that health care workers provide abortion and other reproductive health services because of their moral beliefs not
in spite of them."[48]

The assumption that objecting to abortion care is an issue of conscience
while not recognizing that providing abortion care is also an issue of conscience—
the same assumption that raised concerns for Senator Javits and that is
challenged by providers like Parker—is being amplified by the resources being
deployed through the CRFD by the growing power of a Christian conservative
legal movement led by people like Roger Severino and Jay Sekulow, and through
the conservative media that champions stories like that of the nurse in Vermont.[49]

The HHS website on "Conscience Protections for Healthcare Providers:
describes "Your Conscience Rights" this way: "Conscience protections apply to
health care providers who refuse to perform, accommodate, or assist with certain health care services on religious or moral grounds."[50] Excluded in that conceptualization is the possibility that health care providers might have religious
or moral grounds for providing or participating in those procedures, and that
patients might have religious or moral grounds for seeking them out. The argument that conscience might lead a physician to want to perform an abortion, or
a taxpayer to want to pay for one, or a woman to seek one was an argument that
was lost in the spring of 1973. Losing that argument has not only had concrete
consequences for women—as both the general statistics about declining access
to abortion and the particular story about Kathleen Prieskorn make clear—but
has also flattened out the real-life stories of how conscience is experienced.

Let's return to that case in Vermont. If UVMMC cannot persuade the CRFD
that their policies comply with the Church Amendment, the hospital risks losing $1.6 million dollars in federal funding. In explaining the hospital's efforts
to uphold the Church Amendment's requirements while also meeting their primary obligations to their patients, Dr. Steven Leffler, the interim director of
UVMMC, describes himself as "sympathetic and understanding of our employees and staff who wrestle with their personal beliefs and the demands of their
profession" and makes clear that "anyone employed by UVM Medical Center
may request to be excused from procedures that go against their ethical and religious beliefs." But he adds this as well: "As the state's only academic, tertiary

care center, the world can change in seconds and in the face of all of our best laid staffing plans. Our policy takes into account these situations—and above all else, when there are no other staffing options, our obligation is to our patient."[51]

This particular case, which is still in the process of being resolved, raises more questions than it answers. We know very little, for example, about the nurse who filed the complaint. We know that UVMMC had only recently begun providing elective abortions, a policy that the hospital describes as recommended by the medical staff and unanimously supported by the board of trustees.[52] We don't know, though, how the nurse felt about this policy change or whether she had been included in the discussions leading up to the change. We know that the UVMMC's Fanny Allen Campus in Colchester, which is owned by Covenant Health, a Catholic regional health delivery network, would remain compliant with the Catholic Ethical and Religious Directives and would not be required to provide abortions.[53] We don't know if this particular nurse had tried to move her job four miles away to that campus, where she would have been guaranteed not to have to participate in abortions. Would it be reasonable to expect that of her? We know that she feared losing her job if she refused to assist the doctor. Is acting on that fear the same thing as being compelled to participate in an abortion? We don't know how this nurse's complaint got the attention of the lawyers at the ACLJ and then made its way to the CFRD. Had she been following the political debate on this issue for the past several years? Should her politics matter in assessing the question of whether the hospital violated the Church Amendment?

We know even less about the patient in this case. We know she arrived at the hospital for a legal procedure with the expectation that she would be taken care of by professional health care providers, but we don't know the circumstances that brought her to the hospital that day. Was this an emergency procedure? Had something gone wrong in a planned pregnancy, or was this pregnancy unwanted from the outset? Why was she undergoing the procedure in a hospital, where nationally only 4 percent of abortions take place?[54] Was she aware that her nurse had to be pressured to assist in the procedure and was only doing so out of fear of losing her job? Does she know that her procedure is currently the subject of this legal and political battle?

Different readers will, I imagine, think differently about the significance and relevance of these questions. But asking them matters. These questions remind us that the conscience wars that take place in regulatory procedures, legal battles, political rhetoric, and media discourse also take place in real time, in hospitals, in workplaces, and in people's lives. Focusing only on the former makes certain claims of conscience louder and more legible than others and obscures the complexities of lived experiences. Representative Bella Abzug and Senator Jacob Javits understood that in 1973, and health care providers like Willie Parker, Lisa Harris, and Monica McLemore remind us of that today.

Notes

1. Laurie Goodstein, "Religious Right Believes Donald Trump Will Deliver on His Promises," *New York Times*, November 11, 2016, https://www.nytimes.com/2016 /11/12/us/donald-trump-evangelical-christians-religious-conservatives.html; Emma Green, "The Religious Liberty Show-Downs Coming in 2017," *Atlantic*, December 28, 2016, https://www.theatlantic.com/politics/archive/2016/12/the-religious-liberty -showdowns-coming-in-2017/511400/; Emma Green, "Health and Human Services and the Religious-Liberty War," *Atlantic*, May 7, 2019, https://www.theatlantic.com/politics /archive/2019/05/hhs-trump-religious-freedom/588697/. Also see the section on "The First Amendment and Religious Freedom," in *Republican Party Platform 2016* (Committee on Arrangements for the 2016 Republican National Convention [Cleveland]), https://prod-cdn-static.gop.com/media/documents/DRAFT_12_FINAL%5B1%5D-ben _1468872234.pdf.

2. Exec. Order No. 13,798, (May 4, 2017), "Promoting Free Speech and Religious Liberty," *Federal Register* 82, no. 88 (May 9, 2017): 21675–21676. U.S. Department of Health and Human Services, Office for Civil Rights, "HHS Announces New Conscience and Religious Freedom Division," January 18, 2018, https://web.archive.org /web/20180119180204/https://www.hhs.gov/about/news/2018/01/18/hhs-ocr -announces-new-conscience-and-religious-freedom-division.html; 42 U.S. Code § 300gg–13, Coverage of Preventive Health Services, July 1, 1944, ch. 373, title XXVII, § 2713, as added Pub. L. 111–148, title I, § 1001(5), Mar. 23, 2010, 124 Stat. 131, https://www.law.cornell.edu/uscode/text/42/300gg-13.

3. U.S. Department of Health & Human Services, Office for Civil Rights, "HHS Announces Final Conscience Rule Protecting Health Care Entities and Individuals," May 21, 2019, https://www.hhs.gov/guidance/document/hhs-announces-final -conscience-rule-protecting-health-care-entities-and-individuals. Today, these rules remain at the center of a fight between those who argue that the so-called contraceptive mandate violates the Religious Freedom and Restoration Act (Religious Freedom Restoration Act of 1993, Pub. L. No. 103-141, 107 Stat. 1488, hereafter RFRA) and the Free Exercise rights of those individuals and organizations holding religious objections to some or all forms of contraception, and those who argued that because the mandate represented the government's compelling interest in providing equal and comprehensive preventive care to women it was both constitutional and compliant with RFRA. For a longer discussion of this tension, see Sara Dubow, "'A Constitutional Right Rendered Utterly Meaningless': Religious Exemptions and Reproductive Politics, 1973–2014," *Journal of Policy History* 27, no 1 (2015): 1–35, https://doi.org /10.1017/S0898030614000347.

4. U.S. HHS, Office for Civil Rights, "HHS Announces Final Conscience Rule."

5. U.S. HHS, Office for Civil Rights, "HHS Announces New Conscience and Freedom Protection Division." The HHS OCR had previously focused primarily on the enforcement of Title VII of the Civil Rights Act of 1964, the Americans with Disabilities Act of 1990, and other related federal statutes, as well as enforcing the health information privacy protections of the Health Insurance Portability and Accountability Act (HIPAA).

6. U.S. Department of Health and Human Services, Office for Civil Rights, "Justification of Estimates for Appropriations Committees," in *Fiscal Year 2020*, 36, https://www.hhs.gov/sites/default/files/fy-2020-cj-compilation.pdf.

7. U.S. Department of Health and Human Services, Office for Civil Rights, "Justification of Estimates for Appropriations Committees," in *Fiscal Year 2019*, 28, https://www.hhs.gov/sites/default/files/fy19-departmental-management-cj-4-10-18.pdf.

8. Church Amendment, 42 U.S.C. § 300a-7 (1973).

9. Letter from American Center from Law and Justice to the U.S. Department of Health and Human Services, Conscience and Religious Freedom Division, May 9, 2018, http://media.aclj.org/pdf/ACLJ_OCR_Cmplt_VT.pdf.

10. Letter from American Center from Law and Justice, May 9, 2018.

11. U.S. Department of Health and Human Services, Office for Civil Rights, Conscience and Religious Freedom Division, response to redacted recipient at McDermott Will & Emery LLP, August 28, 2019, https://www.hhs.gov/sites/default/files/uvmmc-nov-letter_508.pdf.

12. Jay Sekulow, "ACLJ Vindicates Rights of Vermont Nurse Who Was Unlawfully Forced to Participate in Abortion—HHS Threatens to Pull Medical Center Funding," press release, August 28, 2019, https://aclj.org/pro-life/aclj-vindicates-rights-of-vermont-nurse-who-was-unlawfully-forced-to-participate-in-abortion-hhs-threatens-to-pull-medical-center-funding.

13. Dennis Carter, "HHS Launches Another Attack on Abortion Providers Under Guise of 'Conscience Rights,'" August 29, 2019, https://rewire.news/article/2019/08/29/hhs-launches-another-attack-on-abortion-providers-under-guise-of-conscience-rights/.

14. Public Law 93–94. 93rd Congress, S. 1136.

15. *Congressional Record* 119, part 8 (March 26, 1973, to April 2, 1973), vote recorded on S9604, March 27, 1973; *Congressional Record* 119, part 35 (January 3, 1973, to December 22, 1973), vote recorded on H17463, May 31, 1973; *Congressional Record* 119, part 35 (January 3, 1973, to December 22, 1973), vote recorded on S18072, June 5, 1973. The only senator to vote against the amendment was William Fulbright (Democrat from Arkansas). He didn't speak during the debate, and his papers don't have any clues that would explain his opposition.

16. Rachel Benson Gold, "Conscience Makes a Comeback in the Age of Managed Care," *Guttmacher Policy Review* 1, no. 1 (1998), https://www.guttmacher.org/gpr/1998/02/conscience-makes-comeback-age-managed-care. According to a 1997 analysis by the Alan Guttmacher Institute, half enacted parallel laws by the end of 1974; by the end of 1978, nearly all states had done so. Statistics available at http://www.guttmacher.org/pubs/tgr/01/1/gr010101.html.

17. In one article, "Clean Air, Solid Waste Acts Extended," *Washington Post*, March 28, 1973, A2, the conscience clause was referenced in one paragraph, and it focused on Nixon's opposition to the bill. *Los Angeles Times*, "The Nation: Senate OK's Right Not to Perform Abortions," March 28, 1973, C2, included one paragraph on the conscience clause in their list of six stories of national interest, including an upcoming Frank Sinatra concert.

18. David M. Alperin, "Abortion and the Law," *Newsweek*, March 3, 1975, 26.

19. For review of that literature, see Dubow, "'Constitutional Right."

20. Thomas M. Messner, "From Culture Wars to Conscience Wars: Emerging Threats to Conscience," No. 2543, Heritage Foundation, April 13, 2011, https://www.heritage.org/civil-society/report/culture-wars-conscience-wars-emerging-threats-conscience.

21. Reva Siegel and Linda Greenhouse, "Before (and After) *Roe v. Wade*: New Questions about Backlash," *Yale Law Journal* 128 (2011), 2031, 2067–2068, https://www.yalelawjournal.org/pdf/987_s9ytqjum.pdf. Republicans like Bob Packwood, Henry Kissinger, George H. W. Bush, Charles Percy, Nelson Rockefeller, and Ronald Reagan all supported abortion reform and legalization.

22. Linda Greenhouse, "Misconceptions," *New York Times*, January 23, 2013, https://web.archive.org/web/20130302132253/https://opinionator.blogs.nytimes.com/2013/01/23/misconceptions/.

23. Letter from Representative Bella Abzug to Joan Dixon, June 25, 1973. In Bella Abzug Papers, Box 600, folder on Abortion Correspondence, 1973, from Rare Book and Manuscript Library, Columbia University, New York City, NY.

24. Lisa Young, *Feminists and Party Politics* (Ann Arbor: University of Michigan Press, 2000); Kira Sanbonmatsu, *Democrats, Republicans, and the Politics of Women's Place* (Ann Arbor: University of Michigan Press, 2002); David Karol, *Party Position Change in American Politics: Coalition Management* (Cambridge: Cambridge University Press, 2003); Catherine Rymph, *Republican Women: Feminism and Conservatism from Suffrage to the Rise of the New Right* (Chapel Hill: University of North Carolina Press, 2009). For a legislative history of the 93rd Congress's actions on women's issues, see Morrigen Holcomb, "Legislation Affecting the Rights of Women Enacted by, or Pending in, the 93rd Congress," *Congressional Research Service*, May 23, 1974; Karen M. Kaufmann and John R. Petrocik, "The Changing Politics of American Men: Understanding the Sources of the Gender Gap," *American Journal of Political Science* 43, no. 3 (1999): 864–887, https://doi.org/10.2307/2991838.

25. Donald Matthews and Jane Sherron De Hart, *Sex, Gender, and the Politics of ERA: A State, and the Nation* (New York: Oxford University Press, 1990); Donald T. Critchlow, *Phyllis Schlafly and Grassroots Conservatism: A Woman's Crusade* (Princeton, NJ: Princeton University Press, 2007). House vote recorded in *Congressional Record* 117, part 28 (October 14, 1971, to October 21, 1971), 35815; Senate vote recorded in *Congressional Record* 118, part 29 (January 18, 1972, to October 18, 1972), 9598.

26. See Morrigene Holcomb, "Legislation Affecting the Rights of Women Enacted by, or Pending in, the 93rd Congress," *Congressional Research Service Report*, May 23, 1974.

27. Letter from Representative Bella Abzug to Joan Dixon, June 25, 1973. In Bella Abzug Papers, Box 600, folder on Abortion Correspondence, 1973, from Rare Book and Manuscript Library, Columbia University, New York City, NY.

28. *Congressional Record* 119, part 35 (January 3, 1973, to December 22, 1973), May 31, 1973, 17452; *Simkins v. Moses H. Cone Memorial Hospital*, 323 F. 2d 959 (4th Circuit, 1963); *Sams v. Valley General Hospital Association*, 413 F. 2d 826 (4th Circuit, 1969).

29. *Congressional Record* 119, May 31, 1973, 17452; *Simkins v. Moses H. Cone Memorial Hospital*; *Sams v. Valley General Hospital Association*.

30. *Congressional Record* 119, May 31, 1973, 17452; *Simkins v. Moses H. Cone Memorial Hospital*; *Sams v. Valley General Hospital Association*.

31. Letter from Brenda Feigen Fasteau, Coordinator, Women's Rights Project, ACLU, to Representative Mr. Marlin D. Schneider, August 28, 1973, cc'd to Bella Abzug, Bella Abzug Papers, Box 605, folder on Abortion Correspondence, 1973, from Rare Book and Manuscript Library, Columbia University, New York City, NY; Letter from National Association for Repeal of Abortion Laws, undated, Bella Abzug Papers, Box 605, folder on Abortion Organizations, NARAL, 1973. Letter from American

Association of University Women to Honorable Bella S. Abzug, November 16, 1973; letter from National Board of the Young Women's Christian Association to Member of Congress, September 1, 1973; letter from Catholics for a Free Choice to Congressperson, November 27, 1973, Bella Abzug Papers; Letter from Eleanor Marvin, President of National Council of Jewish Women, to Representative Harley O. Staggers, May 15, 1973, cc'd to Bella Abzug, Bella Abzug Papers, all from Box 602, folder on Abortion: General.

32. Letter from Representative James F. Hastings to Representative Bella Abzug, May 31, 1973, Bella Abzug Papers, Box 600, folder on Abortion Correspondence, 1973, from Rare Book and Manuscript Library, Columbia University, New York City, NY.

33. Harriet F. Pilpel and Dorothy E. Patton, "Abortion, Conscience, and the Constitution: An Examination of Federal Institutional Conscience Clauses," *Columbia Human Rights Law Review* 6, no. 2: (1974–1975): 279–305.

34. Letter from Robert F. Drinan to Ms. Pamela Lowry, June 11, 1973, Harriet F. Pilpel Papers, Sophia Smith Collection, Smith College, Northampton, MA.

35. Morrigene Holcomb, "Legislation Affecting the Rights of Women Enacted by, or Pending in, the 93rd Congress," Congressional Research Service, HG 1428 U.S.D.,74-109GGR, May 23, 1974, https://digital.library.unt.edu/ark:/67531/metadc1229497/; Morrigene Holcomb and Karen Keesling, "Women's Rights Legislation in the 94th Congress," Congressional Research Service, 77-36G, February 9, 1977, https://digital.library.unt.edu/ark:/67531/metadc1229299/.

36. Letter from Betz Christianson to Representative Bella Abzug, September 27, 1973, in Bella Abzug Papers, Box 600, folder on Abortion Correspondence, 1973, from Rare Book and Manuscript Library, Columbia University, New York City, NY.

37. Rachel K. Jones, Elizabeth Witwer, and Jenna Jerman, *Abortion Incidence and Service Availability in the United States, 2017* (New York: Guttmacher Institute, 2019), https://doi.org/10.1363/2019.30760.

38. Dan Keating, Tim Meko, and Danielle Rindler, "Abortion Access Is More Difficult for Women in Poverty," *Washington Post*, July 10, 2019, https://www.washingtonpost.com/national/2019/07/10/abortion-access-is-more-difficult-women-poverty/.

39. Elaine L. Hill, David Slutsky, and Donna Ginther, "Reproductive Health Care in Catholic-Owned Hospitals," National Bureau of Economic Research, NBER Working Paper Series, February 2016, 10, https://www.nber.org/papers/w23768.

40. Molly M. Ginty, "Treatment Denied," *Ms.* Blog, May 9, 2011, https://msmagazine.com/blog/blog/2011/05/09/treatment-denied/.

41. Senator Jacob Javits (R-NY). "Public Health Service Extension Act." *Congressional Record* 119, Part 35 (January 3, 1973, to December 22, 1973), March 27, 1973, S9599 and S9603.

42. Letter from Caroline Kennedy to Representative Bella Abzug, April 17, 1973, in Bella Abzug Papers, Box 600, folder on Abortion Correspondence, 1973, from Rare Book and Manuscript Library, Columbia University, New York City, NY.

43. Jimmye Kimmey, "Right to Choose Memorandum, Schlesinger Library, Radcliffe Institute for Advanced Study, Harvard University, NARAL Collection, MC 313, box 6 ("ASA" file), reprinted in Greenhouse and Siegel, *Before Roe v. Wade*, 33.

44. For earlier work on this issue, see Carol Joffe, *Doctors of Conscience: The Struggle to Provide Abortion before and after Roe v. Wade* (Boston: Beacon Press, 1995). For more recent arguments, see Mara Buchbinder, Dragana Lassiter, Rebecca Mercier, Amy Bryant, and Anne Drapkin Lyerly, "Reframing Conscientious Care: Providing Abortion Care When Law and Conscience Collide," *Hastings Center Report* 46, no. 2 (2016):

22–30, https://doi.org/10.1002/hast.545; Lisa H. Harris, "Recognizing Conscience in Abortion Provision," *New England Journal of Medicine* 367, no. 11 (2012): 981–983, https://doi.org/10.1056/nejmp1206253.

45. Willie Parker, *Life's Work: From the Trenches, A Moral Argument for Choice* (New York: 37Ink, 2017).

46. Quote is from Willie Parker, "Personal Jesus," *Conscience Magazine*, August 22, 2016, https://www.catholicsforchoice.org/resource-library/personal-jesus-3/.

47. Harris, "Recognizing Conscience," 982.

48. Monica R. McLemore, "If You Don't Want to Provide Abortions, Don't Go into Health-care," *Vice*, September 3, 2019, https://www.vice.com/en_us/article/9kead5/vermont-abortion-nurse-if-you-dont-want-to-provide-abortions-dont-go-into-healthcare.

49. Daniel Bennett, *Defending Faith: The Politics of the Christian Legal Movement* (Lawrence: University of Kansas Press, 2017); Scott A. Merriman, *When Religious and Secular Interests Collide: Faith, Law, and the Religious Exemption Debate* (Santa Barbara, CA: Praeger, 2017); Steven M. Teles, *The Rise of the Conservative Legal Movement* (Princeton, NJ: Princeton University Press, 2008); Jefferson Decker, *The Other Rights Revolution: Conservative Lawyers and the Remaking of American Government* (New York: Oxford University Press, 2016).

50. U.S. Department of Health and Human Services, "Conscience Protections for Health Care Providers," https://web.archive.org/web/20190929095823/https://www.hhs.gov/conscience/conscience-protections/index.html.

51. Stephen Leffler, "Religious Beliefs and Medical Care," *VTDigger*, September 2, 2019, https://vtdigger.org/2019/09/02/stephen-leffler-religious-beliefs-and-medical-care/.

52. Dan D'Ambrosio, "UVM Medical Center Reverses Policy; Will Provide Elective Abortions," *Burlington Free Press*, January 25, 2018, https://www.burlingtonfreepress.com/story/news/2018/01/25/uvm-medical-center-reverses-policy-provide-elective-abortions/1059921001/. This was a change in a policy that had existed since 1972 that the hospital only provided abortions in cases of medical necessity.

53. D'Ambrosio, "UVM Medical Center."

54. Jones et al., "Abortion Incidence."

Chapter 7

Abortion as an Act of Conscience

Curtis Boyd and Glenna Halvorson-Boyd

The public debate that swirls around legal abortion centers on two questions. First, is it morally acceptable to end an embryonic or fetal life? Second, do we as a society entrust the pregnant woman with that moral decision? The first question takes the developing pregnancy as its focus, while the second focuses on the moral agency of the woman.

We typically fail to link the two questions in our public discourse. In our highly politicized debate, those who oppose abortion focus solely on the first question, to which they have an absolute answer (typically grounded in religious beliefs): "No! Never." Therefore the second question is moot. The woman has no rights and thus no standing in the matter. Those who support abortion rights appear to focus only on the second question, asserting the woman's legal right to sovereignty over her own body. Thus, the two "sides" talk past each other, arguing not different points of view but different points, thereby appearing to dismiss the other's question. In the United States, the "debate" has devolved into a virtual holy war in which the truth of women's experience and that of abortion providers is lost in battle.

We speak to the issue as a team who has devoted the past fifty years to securing and providing legal abortions in the United States: Curtis Boyd as a physician and Glenna Halvorson-Boyd as a psychologist. The words and the spirit we bring to our work are something we have created together.

Our paths to this work were very different. Curtis grew up in a deeply religious community in rural east Texas. His beloved grandmother, MaMa Boyd, believed he had a special mission from God and he was "called" while still in high school to preach. At university he was shocked to learn that the Bible had not been originally written in the English of King James. That revelation and other experiences of a world larger than the farms and fields of his childhood led him to question the fundamentalist Christianity of his early years. Curtis longed for a religion of compassion and inclusion, and in medical school he joined the Unitarian Church which met this need. His family was forever disappointed that he chose a career in medicine over his calling into the ministry.

Glenna's journey from her childhood and family to the work of psychology in abortion care was neither as long nor as unexpected as Curtis's. She grew up in suburban California, raised by a devoutly atheist father who maintained that much of the evil in the world was done in the name of one religion or another, and a mother who was an agnostic and stressed the importance of both individual conscience and social conscience. Both of her parents were feminists in word and deed. Her mother had a career, and her father did more of the cooking. Glenna was expected to pursue a meaningful career and to do her part to make the world a better place, so working for social change was expected. However, the simple fact of being female gave the work added meaning. As a young woman becoming sexually active, Glenna lived with the fear of an ill-timed pregnancy. And the insults of her mother's gynecologist when she requested a prescription for the newly available birth control pill while she was unmarried stayed in her mind. She prevailed and got the pill.

From these very different backgrounds we each became active in the civil rights movement of the 1960s and the women's rights movement of the late 1960s and early 1970s—a natural progression for Glenna; an awakening for Curtis.

Through the Unitarian Church, Curtis met ministers who were working with the Clergy Consultation Service on Problem Pregnancy to find safe places to refer women for abortion care. These ministers asked Curtis to assist in the search—which proved fruitless. Frustrated and knowing Curtis was committed to the concept of safe abortion for women, the ministers asked if he would provide abortions himself. In 1968 Curtis began to provide illegal abortions secretly within his existing family practice.

Most of his abortion patients were referred through the Clergy Consultation Service. Curtis recognized that women who received counsel from the ministers were better prepared for the physical and emotional experience of abortion. He also realized that as a physician he was neither trained nor qualified to provide such counsel. Thus, when abortion became legal with the 1973 Supreme Court decision, Curtis opened the first legal abortion clinic in Texas, and one of his priorities was to provide abortion counseling. He recruited Glenna to train the first group of legal abortion counselors in the southwest.

Glenna developed an individual counseling protocol grounded in the fact that the pregnancy and the decision to continue or end it occur within the context of the woman's life. Appreciating the context and thus the meaning of the decision for each patient requires active listening on the part of all staff, particularly in the preabortion counseling session. Our approach is informed by existential theory with its emphasis on choice, freedom, responsibility, anxiety, and the search for meaning. As we listen carefully to each woman's story, we find it is typically an exploration of her moral decision-making process.

Although our patients seldom frame their efforts to do the best thing at a difficult time in their lives as a moral quest, their stories tell us that it has been and will continue to be an exploration of their morality and ethics. A patient wrote of her decision to end her pregnancy in one of the journals we keep in our recovery room:

> Today is a day I never saw coming. Nowhere in my life did I ever think I'd be here making one of the toughest decisions in my life, but I myself know what will be the best for me as much as it hurts. I know I'll recover from this and move on. I'll know how hard it is to go through something that you never see coming. I know I'll always live with this guilt but I pray to my savior to help me in life to continue.

Neither of us intended to make abortion our life work. We imagined that the abortion clinic was a temporary measure, a way to meet the need until abortion became a routine part of medical practice. Obviously, we were wrong. Abortion has remained a subspecialty, most often provided in a clinic setting. The harassment and violence against abortion providers, which began in 1980, continues today as a routine part of daily life. The continued violence against abortion providers is, in fact, a large part of why abortion has not been absorbed into the mainstream of U.S. medicine. When we walk through a hostile crowd shouting "Murderers!" we understand why other doctors, nurses, and counselors do not choose to openly provide abortions.

We have always approached our work as an affirmation of life—both the woman's life and the life she wishes for a child she would bear. In doing so, we place value on the pregnancy, and we respect the moral agency of the pregnant woman. For us as for most of our patients, their sovereignty and their concern for their fetus are *not* abstract; both are real, pressing, and sometimes painful. One of our patients put it this way: "Despite this decision being the most difficult I have ever made, I know with all my heart that it was the best for myself and my little one." Then she writes directly to her aborted fetus:

Little baby, someday I know you will return to me to see your sweet smile
and hope giving eyes. And that day you will know a father that loves you
more than the world and you will be given a chance for a healthy and
prosperous life. You were a precious gift and a major awakening at the
perfect time in my life. Already we have shared laughter and tears and
a plethora of sadness, joy, and fears. Enjoy the timeless love of the universe, my dear. I will see you soon when it's right for you here.

She signs her note, "With all the love I possess."

In performing abortions, we are confronted daily with the reality of both
the pregnant woman's life and the developing embryo or fetus. We have intimate working knowledge of embryonic and fetal development and thus no illu-
sions about what we are doing. Similarly, most women who have abortions in
the United States already have one or more children, and those who do not
imagine that one day they will. All recognize that the fetus is alive and that continuing a pregnancy is a real and enduring commitment.

We contend based on fifty years of listening to women as they struggle with
or state with clarity the decision to continue or terminate a pregnancy that pregnant women have high regard for the fetus. They seldom engage in denial of
the magnitude of the life decision they are making. They regularly show us pho-
tos of their children and talk about their children as the center of their lives.
This occurs as they are simultaneously deciding to end the current fetal life—
in order to care for the children they already have, to pursue important life goals,
or to become capable of mothering children in the future. It is because they care
so deeply about the quality of both their existent and potential children's lives
that they choose abortion.

One Christmas we received a card from a former patient. It read "Peace on
Earth," and she wrote,

Dear Dr. Boyd, in 1973 you gave me an abortion. I was 26 years old, new
in town, waiting tables. I am now 42 with two boys 4 & 9. Although both
of their fathers left when I was pregnant, I was ready to love, nurture and
support them. I often think how different it would have been had my
abortion been impossible. I don't know which would have been worse—
being a confused, inadequate, impoverished mother, twisting my soul to
give the baby away, or experiencing an illegal abortion. I'm especially
grateful to doctors like you. I'm sure you take a lot of flak and see a lot of
troubled women. But you make it possible for so many women to have
healthy families. Thank you and Merry Christmas.

She enclosed a photo of herself and two smiling boys.

We believe that for years the pro-choice movement in the United States has denied the value of the fetus and has done so to our detriment. We sound insensitive, uncaring, and out of touch with reality when we speak only of the woman's right. To recognize the fetus and its value and our own often tender feelings is to be human and humane, and it need not undermine the woman's sovereign right to make the moral decision.

Whether it is morally acceptable to end an embryonic or fetal life is a matter of individual conscience, and we believe the only person qualified to make that decision is the pregnant woman. The women we see accept that solemn responsibility. As one of our patients wrote in our journal to other patients she imagined had or would struggle as she had, "You are human and that requires making difficult choices, even choices you don't like."

Curtis faced his own decision of conscience fifty years ago and obviously decided that he had a moral responsibility to provide abortions. Curtis's path to that decision makes clear the moral—and in his case religious—roots that often support the decision to have or provide an abortion. Women, too, understood that their religious beliefs helped them to decide for an abortion and thanked God for guiding them through the process. "I have been praying and praying and we went over so many options to have the baby," one woman wrote. "However, the cons outweighed the pros by a mile. Thank you Lord for giving me the team of doctors and nurses that you did. They were so kind and gentle. Thank you Lord for helping me find this facility."

Women who come to us for abortion care may not see themselves as engaged in an ethical decision-making process demonstrating a high level of moral development. But they are, and we are aware of it every day. We see a woman who knows she cannot be a good mother at this time: she is too immature (her words, not ours), she lives in poverty, she is drug addicted, or she is in an abusive relationship in which she and her children are not safe. These women may have children now and want other children in the future, when they believe they can be good mothers, provide a family and community of support, and realize some of their own dreams and aspirations. As one patient explains her decision to the fetus she is aborting,

> I came in today loving you . . . so small and already [I am] so in love. For-
> give me my little one. I am 19 years old with a 10-month-old already.
> I would have loved to be your mommy and to have been able to love you
> the way I do your brother, but he still needs so much of me—of my

attention. I'm not ready for you baby. Give me time, for God will send you back to me.

Women have abortions because they want to be good mothers. The fetus has value to the pregnant woman, and it has value to us. But the fetus does not have equal value, nor should it have rights equal to or superseding those of the pregnant woman. The abortion issue must focus on the full personhood of the woman. As the last patient statement makes clear, the woman considers the potential personhood of the fetus in terms of her psychological state, personal history, social situation, and the meaning and implications of this pregnancy for everyone's future. The pregnant woman reflects upon what is good for the creation of which she is an agent. Pregnant women are not only capable of moral decision making; fortunately, they make moral decisions every day. And those of us who do this work have the honor of bearing witness.

Bearing witness is an old religious concept, and our experience underscores the importance of religion, not only in Curtis's life but in the lives and decision-making of most of our patients and their families, and in the history of the movement for reproductive justice. The strongest institutional support for abortion reform and then abortion rights in the United States came from religious groups.

We want to close with a family story. It is no surprise that Glenna's parents were always extremely supportive of our work while Curtis's family mostly looked the other way. They knew but never spoke of it. Glenna never met Curtis's grandmother, MaMa Boyd, as she was already dead when we met. However, when Curtis spoke of her, it was with love and pain. He knew that he had disappointed her—that she had died hoping he would one day "come home preaching Jesus Christ and him crucified." Then NBC News did a story on Curtis as the most unlikely of abortion providers, given his small-town roots and religious background. We showed the piece to his immediate family—some of them were interviewed in it. As images of their hometown, the farm, the family burial ground filled the TV screen, his brother-in-law stage whispered, "You think you're so special! You're not the first person in this family to do abortions. Bet you didn't know your MaMa Boyd did abortions when she was a midwife."

We had not known that Curtis's beloved grandmother with her deep religious faith had done this same work before he was ever born. She no doubt acted from compassion and mercy. Those values and the injunction to "love thy neighbor as thyself"—to treat others with the dignity and respect we wish for ourselves—inform most of the world's faith traditions and, as in Glenna's case, moral teachings. Both patients and providers experience abortion as an act of conscience.

Chapter 8

The Meaning of Viability in Abortion Care

Shelley Sella

I started providing abortion care in 1990 and around ten years later, I met Dr. George Tiller, who was known worldwide for providing abortion care later in pregnancy. I was mentored by and worked with Dr. Tiller at his clinic in Wichita, Kansas, for seven years, providing abortion care throughout pregnancy. Following his assassination in 2009, my colleague, Dr. Susan Robinson, and I began providing abortion care in Albuquerque, New Mexico, at Southwestern Women's Options.

Until now, the State of New Mexico has not placed restrictions on nor banned postviable abortions, and we have not been constrained by issues of fetal viability. However, in 2013 there was an initiative on the ballot to ban abortions after twenty weeks in the City of Albuquerque. Thanks to broad-based community support, this initiative was soundly defeated.

We see two groups of patients who come later in pregnancy. Those who are ending a pregnancy because there is something very wrong with their baby—and the word "baby" is the term they invariably use—are known in practice as "fetal indications" patients, and we have no gestational limit for these patients. The second group, "maternal indications," come because of severe challenges and complications in their life or their family's life. We see these patients electively to thirty-two weeks' gestational age and after that on a case-by-case basis. We are thus spared telling most extremely desperate women the bad news that they will be forced to continue their pregnancy.

That being said, the issue of viability is still an important one to me. I believe that *all* abortions that we perform in our practice, and not just after twenty-four weeks when viability is *presumed* to occur, are performed for nonviable pregnancies. When a woman rejects her pregnancy, for whatever reason, at whatever gestational age, the pregnancy ceases to be viable to her. She comes to me to terminate her nonviable pregnancy safely and compassionately. This is how I frame the issue of viability.

The *medical definition* of viability of a fetus or unborn child is that it is able to live after birth. This concurs with the Supreme Court's definition in *Colautti v. Franklin*: "Viability is reached when, in the judgment of the attending physician on the particular facts before him, there is a reasonable likelihood of the fetus' sustained survival outside the womb, with or without artificial support."[1] Note that no gestational age is stated, giving latitude in any direction.

The *Roe v. Wade* ruling adds, "For the stage subsequent to viability, the State, in promoting its interest in the potentiality of human life, may, if it chooses, regulate, and even proscribe, abortion except where it is necessary, in appropriate medical judgment, for the preservation of the life or health of the mother."[2]

The concept of artificial support as considered in these cases presents by definition a mechanistic approach to this issue. If we consider a premature baby or one with fetal abnormalities, artificial support could include mechanical ventilation, medications, or multiple surgeries.

Consider a different viewpoint and a different definition of viability, one that fully takes into account the issue of "sustained survival outside the womb, with or without artificial support." The biological definition of viability— "capable of surviving or living successfully, especially under particular environmental conditions"—places viability within a specific context. In the *Roe v. Wade* decision, the State may regulate and even ban postviable abortions except where necessary, in appropriate medical judgment, for the preservation of the life or health of the mother. The *Doe v. Bolton* decision, which accompanies *Roe v. Wade*, elucidates the concept of medical judgment. "The medical judgment may be exercised in light of all factors—physical, emotional, psychological, familial, and the woman's age—relevant to the wellbeing of the patient. All these factors may relate to health. This allows the attending physician the room he needs to make his best medical judgment. And it is room that operates for the benefit, not the disadvantage, of the pregnant woman."[3]

It is the *Doe v. Bolton* decision that informs my abortion practice in all trimesters, but especially for those in the third trimester. However, the two decisions, *Roe v. Wade* and *Doe v. Bolton* posit potentially opposing interests: the fetus with its potentiality for viability and the woman, who is the patient. The physician is given the power to be the arbiter—to weigh the factors that a woman considers when she decides whether or not to continue a pregnancy and whether or not she considers her pregnancy viable. In contrast to artificial support,

I would call this life support. Life support includes, but is not limited to, adequate food, shelter, financial resources, adequate maturity, safety, health of the mother and the baby both during the pregnancy and after birth, family, community support, and finally love. And yet, even with all of these factors in place, a woman may know that having a child at this time is not right for her and she will still pursue an abortion.

Our patients have a clear-eyed view of their lives and are realistic about their capabilities of caring for a child. Here are some quotes from journals that patients haven written in after their abortion. One patient said, "The way I think of it is my baby is in a better place. This world is evil and full of awful things, not a place to bring an innocent child into." Another said, "My dear baby. I am sorry I have forsaken you. I pray that you will have a beautiful life up in the heavens. One much more abundant than what I can offer you. I really do love you. Rest in peace, Mommy." A fetal indications patient whose baby had severe hydrocephalous said, "I wouldn't have wanted my mom to bring me into the world like that and I can't see doing that to another human being."[4] These are some of the questions that women consider when deciding whether their pregnancy is viable or not.

- For fetal indications: What disabilities will my baby have? What medical interventions will be necessary for its survival? And what impact will those interventions have on its future life? What impact will the abnormalities have on my baby, on me, on my partner, and on my other children? What will be the financial burden on my family?
- For maternal indications: What kind of home environment will this child come into? Is it safe? Will having this baby tie me down with an abusive partner? What are my financial resources? Will my age affect my ability to parent adequately? Will having a baby at my age impact my educational opportunities? Will I be able to finish middle school, or high school, or go to college? How will having a baby affect my existing health issues? How will the baby be affected by my addiction?

Here are examples of two patients who both made the decision that their pregnancies were nonviable. The first patient delivered her first, very wanted child at seven months: a stillborn. One year later, she gave birth to a premature infant who survived but had an abnormality that was repaired soon after birth. Subsequently, hydrocephalous, the abnormal accumulation of fluid in the brain, was diagnosed. The baby required twenty surgical procedures to drain the fluid and died when he was one-and-a-half years old. Three years later, she was happily pregnant again; this time, an ultrasound at twenty-six weeks detected hydrocephalous again. As soon as she got the ultrasound results, she scheduled an appointment for an abortion.

The second patient was a young woman, a mother of three. She had been in an abusive relationship with her husband for years. At one point, she was in professional school, but her husband threatened to kill her if she pursued her studies, so she dropped out. When she found out that she was pregnant, she knew right away that the best decision for her, given her situation, was to seek abortion care. But she was held captive by her husband who threatened to kill her if she had an abortion. One day, her husband pulled a gun on her. In the struggle that followed, the police were called, and her husband was taken to jail. It was only then that she could escape to seek abortion care; by then she had passed the gestational age in her state and came to see us.

Women who decide to continue a pregnancy and have their baby adopted view the pregnancy as a viable one, but not for them. The patients that *we* see have considered this option but have rejected it for many reasons. They feel as strongly about adoption as others feel about abortion. If forced to continue the pregnancy, most would not pursue adoption. Their concerns: They worry deeply that their child will grow up feeling abandoned, that it was not wanted. They worry that it will be mistreated. They worry that the child will find them years later and discover, for example, that their mother was raped when she was fifteen. If they are addicted to drugs or alcohol, they worry that their child will be unhealthy and they don't want their child or the adoptive parents to suffer. They worry that their child *won't* be adopted and will grow up "in the system," in sub-optimal foster care. And finally, some patients come from families and communities where adoption is unacceptable and they fear that they will be forced to care for the child.

Even when a woman considers her pregnancy nonviable, I still may not be able to care for her. In addition to the question of viability is the question, Would this procedure be safe to perform in the outpatient setting? My decision to accept a patient is partly based on the belief that I can safely and successfully complete the abortion in the outpatient setting. We recently turned down a patient at twenty-eight weeks; we might otherwise have cared for her, but she had a history of four cesarean deliveries, and we felt it would be unsafe to proceed in the clinic.

When I think of viability, I think of the viability of the pregnancy as the woman sees it. The question of potential fetal survival is only one issue of many, which include the physical, emotional, financial, and spiritual well-being of the child, the mother, and the family. I would argue that *all* abortions that we do in our practice—first, second, and third trimester—are performed for nonviable pregnancies. This understanding, buttressed by the *Doe v. Bolton* decision, provides the framework for my work.

Notes

1. Colautti v. Franklin, 439 U.S. 379 (1979).
2. Roe v. Wade, 410 U.S. 113 (1973).
3. Doe v. Bolton, 410 U.S. 179 (1973).
4. Hydrocephalus, the abnormal accumulation of fluid in the brain, can lead to severe disabilities and a shortened life span.

Chapter 9

Dangertalk

Voices of Abortion Providers

Lisa A. Martin, Jane A. Hassinger,
Michelle Debbink, and Lisa H. Harris

Introduction

A number of researchers have described the difficulties of doing abortion work.[1]
Wendy Simonds's ethnography of abortion clinic workers recounts stories of discomfort with fetal parts and the violence and gruesomeness that is part of providing abortion care.[2] Kathleen Roe found that abortion providers experience considerable ambivalence in their work.[3] Allyson Lipp described how nurses in abortion care sometimes struggle to provide nonjudgmental care, making considerable efforts to conceal judgments from patients.[4] Collectively, this research reveals that abortion providers hold complicated feelings and attitudes about both abortion and the women they serve.[5]

One obvious source of difficulty in doing abortion work is the associated stigma.[6] Abortion is "dirty work"—a socially necessary task or occupation generally regarded by others as physically disgusting, socially degrading, and/or morally dubious.[7] We have previously described the psychosocial costs to individual providers of doing dirty work, including the burdens associated with disclosing their work to others.[8] Many providers routinely choose not to talk about their work publicly. This self-censorship occurs for a range of reasons including the desire to avoid stressful interactions, protect personal safety, and prevent conflict within families.[9]

Sometimes, however, providers also choose to remain silent to protect the pro-choice movement. In her critique of pro-choice rhetoric, Jeannie Ludlow explored how the movement has created a hierarchy of abortion narratives—what she deems the "politically necessary" stories—that advocates routinely deploy to keep abortion legal (e.g., rape, incest, or domestic violence victims).[10]

Also common are the "politically acceptable" narratives (e.g., contraceptive failures and fetal anomalies) that evoke sympathy. Ludlow's third category, "the things we cannot say," includes stories that are both absent from pro-choice discourse and often exploited by antiabortion activists (e.g., multiple abortions, grief after abortion, and the economics of abortion). Providers keep these stories to themselves because they fear providing fodder for antiabortion groups' rhetoric.[11]

Providers who speak out about these topics have, in fact, been labeled as dangerous to the movement. Harris described the violence in abortion and argued that abortion providers cannot ignore the fetus because fetal parts comprise the concrete evidence that they have done their job of ending a pregnancy.[12] Her acknowledgment that providers sometimes have emotional reactions to the fetus' visual impact, corporeality, and moral significance elicited angry responses from both anti- and pro-choice communities, including harassing emails and threats from antiabortion activists who seized upon her words as proof that abortion is gruesome and should be banned. Simultaneously, Lisa Harris was criticized by some pro-choice advocates who felt she should have remained quiet.[13] Providers' experiences may not perfectly align with pro-choice messaging, creating tension between feminist activists and those doing the work that feminists champion.[14]

Few scholars have examined whether providers' self-silencing results in costs to the movement itself. One consequence is that nuanced public depictions of abortion workers are rare. The absence of providers' voices has created a vacuum in which stereotypical caricatures may dominate the public discourse. Both abortion supporters and opponents commonly construct providers in one-dimensional terms: celebrated as "heroes" and "warriors" in the fight for women's reproductive autonomy or vilified as callous, incompetent, and greedy.[15] Some restrictive abortion laws—allegedly designed to protect patients from abortion providers—rely on these negative stereotypes.[16]

Roe, one of the first to document provider ambivalence within abortion, worried that ignoring difficult aspects of abortion work would ultimately weaken the abortion rights movement.[17] She advocated that proponents of safe, legal abortion look to providers' work experiences to help shape more resonant frameworks for understanding and conveying the complexities of abortion. Nearly thirty years later, we answer that call.

Using qualitative data from abortion providers' discussions, we explore tensions between their narratives and the dominant abortion rights discourse and examine the types of stories about which providers routinely remain silent. We seek to understand how providers' self-censorship around the difficult aspects of the work may impact the pro-choice movement and how giving voice to these tensions might transform current abortion discourse. In addition, we consider the broad implications of suppressing dangertalk on social movements.

Methods

We analyzed data from two iterations of the Providers Share Workshop: a pilot study conducted in 2007, and a seven-site study from 2010 to 2012.[18] The workshop is a multisession facilitated intervention in which teams of abortion providers explore their work experiences.[19] The workshop was designed and implemented to create space for conversations about the unique rewards and stresses experienced by abortion workers, including being targets of violence, harassment, and restrictive legislation. Workshop sessions addressed the following themes: (1) what abortion work means to me; (2) stories of memorable patients; (3) abortion and identity; (4) abortion politics; and (5) future directions for self-care. Eligible participants included all workers in abortion care, including counselors, surgical assistants, physicians, nurses, clinic managers, and administrators. There were no substantive changes between the pilot and multisite workshops. The participants provided written, informed consent for participation, audio recording, and publication of deidentified findings.

We recorded and transcribed all sessions. All study team members read the transcripts and identified major themes, using an iterative coding process for reconciling disagreements. Data collected from pilot transcripts were coded using NVivo 8. Transcripts from the second, multisite study were coded using Dedoose. The University of Michigan institutional review board approved both studies.

Results

Ninety-six people at eight clinic sites participated. The workshop sites represented each major US geographic region as well as a variety of service models (freestanding clinics, clinics integrated within health systems, for-profit, and nonprofit). The participants filled a range of job types within abortion care, and we use the term "provider" to mean all of those involved in direct patient care at these sites. The participants were predominantly female.

Here we focus on the stories not routinely shared with friends, family, or even other abortion worker colleagues. Outside the workshops, such stories were typically censored because of concern about affirming antiabortion stereotypes, challenging pro-choice movement messaging, and acknowledging moral ambiguities in abortion work.

Stories We Don't Share

Judging Patients

The providers revealed that they were not immune to negative stereotypes about women seeking abortions, and many admitted that they sometimes judged their patients. In particular, the providers felt ambivalence and expressed that some women are less deserving of an abortion, in particular when they have multiple abortions or refuse to use reliable contraceptive methods:

> She used to come in all the time. . . . She didn't use contraceptives, and they were being offered to her. And she was not a young person. She had . . . seven or eight children. Now she's coming in without using any birth control of any type—a "frequent flier." She comes in [for the] number fifteen abortion. And I just had a little problem with that.

These types of patients failed to evoke providers' empathy. Many participants spoke about the importance of confronting their own negative attitudes, reminding themselves that their job was to provide care, not to judge. The providers also described efforts to conceal judgment from patients—efforts that were not always successful.

Moral Uncertainty

Although the participants often commented about their pride in their work, many also identified moral uncertainties about whether providing abortions was always a good thing. For example, one physician stated,

> I still to this day say to myself I hope I'm doing the right thing. That never goes away. I embrace [this uncertainty] as healthy because . . . it lets me know that certainty about being right is not necessary to move forward. . . . I hope we can talk about [this] because it's one of the most dangerous parts—[the] "of course it's right to do abortions" assumption. But to talk about maybe it's not always right or doesn't always feel right. . . . There's part of this where you need some validation [that] what you're doing is right.

Another physician described her conflicting feelings when administering digoxin to stop the fetal heart in abortions later in pregnancy:

> I don't get to talk about it all the time. But when I was an ob-gyn resident . . . it was terrible when someone came in with a complication because everything in neonatal medicine now is geared toward saving

that twenty-four [week fetus]. . . . Now that I deliver digoxin to twenty-three to twenty-four weekers, it's very difficult. I never enjoyed trying to save a twenty-three-and-a-half [week fetus], but I don't really enjoy giving digoxin . . . either. It's the exact same "yuck."

Religion and Religious Intolerance in Pro-Choice Communities

Many participants spoke about the influence of their religious faith on their work. Some found that abortion work fit well with their Christian values and beliefs:

> I am pro-choice, and I work in abortion care. I am also a very strong Christian and very faith-based. And for a lot of people those don't work. But in myself and my way of thinking, they mesh so perfectly.

Said another,

> Christianity preaches love and acceptance and compassion and empathy. It doesn't preach judgment and anger and shouting and violence. It just doesn't. And I feel like what I do is compassionate. I provide compassionate care for women who need that love and sensitivity and validation in their lives. . . . It's not a conflict inside me at all.

Others expressed resentment that protesters often constitute the only visible face of religious faith when it comes to abortion, thus erasing the compatibility of being religious and supporting abortion.

> It's really hard for me to see the protestors that we get—the religious protestors. Like I said, that phrase that I keep saying just kind of sums it up to me: God wants spiritual fruits, not religious nuts. I feel like the people that stand outside our clinics and protest and say that they do it because of their faith or because of what the Bible says, they are so judgmental. . . . I feel like those protestors give so much fuel to people who are against religion or against Christianity, and that's heartbreaking to me because I don't see my faith as a heavy thing. I see my faith as such an uplifting thing, such a strengthening thing to me. And for people to get that nasty impression of Christians, it just makes me angry.

However, other providers spoke about struggles with reconciling their work with messages about abortion from their churches. "I try to distance myself from that. . . . I think my childhood growing up, eighteen years of Catholic school, it's still hard for me to accept what I do, even though I want to do this . . . and I'm fine with it. There's still this inner struggle sometimes."

In discussing religion, several participants shared that it felt uncomfortable or even dangerous to reveal religious commitments and convictions while at work. Because the conservative religious movement is viewed by many abortion workers as the opposition, they feared potential tensions among colleagues. One shared,

> It's a thing that I deal with within myself every day because I am a practicing Muslim—that I represent the religious right or something—or a group of people that are considered the enemy in abortion care and abortion work. I don't know how I feel about that. . . . I guess I feel little bit like I don't want to be the token . . . religious person who feels differently about abortion. . . . I do believe in God, I pray, and I practice these tenets of life, and that's OK . . . so I guess for me politics/religion they are a hand-in-hand thing.

Another expressed surprise at the level of religious intolerance within the clinic: "I came from a very spiritual base when I came here. And I couldn't believe the intolerance . . . in [this organization]."

Fulfilling Antiabortion Stereotypes

The providers worried that they might sometimes resemble the antiabortion caricatures of providers as callous, uncaring "butchers" who killed babies and injured women. One person shared a story about struggling with overwhelming numbers of patients, feeling that she indeed worked in what the antiabortion groups would call an "abortion mill": "It's like a slaughterhouse—it's like—line 'em up and kill 'em and then go on to the next one—I feel like that sometimes."

Other providers worried that they caused their patients pain. For various reasons, a woman's anesthesia may be inadequate during her abortion. Providers worried that patients' experience of pain could color their perceptions of providers and the work. "Doing the work may cause people pain; they are screaming in agony, but we just do what we do. In any other situation [it] would be considered torture, but we do it, and you know all of us just kind of pack it away."

A male participant noted that he worked to combat stereotypes of men as unfeeling: "My role is shaped a great deal by my biology, by virtue of being a man doing this work and of having a very real need to avoid the perception of being a torturer." Participants acknowledged that sometimes they must ignore a patient's physical discomfort in order to complete the procedure. "It's sort of basically that I have to get the procedure done; I can't stop and say, 'Oh, I'm sorry I'm hurting you, and do you need a minute?' You know, you just have to get it done."

Fears that a patient's experience could lead to "setbacks" in abortion access amplified providers' worry about fulfilling negative stereotypes. Said one clinician,

> [I'm] aware that any bad experience could set us back so much . . . if . . . people talk about it and . . . tell people how bad it is, and how you can get hurt from it. . . . I feel like it's part of my responsibility in some f-cked up way to make sure that I help keep abortions going.

Life and Death Encounters with Fetuses

For many providers, considering whether they view abortion as killing presents a particularly challenging dilemma. One provider described how her work is similar to being a soldier: "[Abortion work] feels like being in war. . . . I think about what soldiers feel like when they kill." Another observed,

> Abortion is life and death, and I think for me it's about providers saying, "Yes, we end lives here," and being okay with that. Because I feel like a lot of us may have different opinions. . . . I had a woman wake up in the recovery room and say, "I just killed my baby." And I said to her, "You did, and that's okay." And just, being okay, to say that. And we don't all agree with that's what we're doing here. But that's what I feel we're doing here. And I'm okay with that.

Said one, as she contemplated antiabortion protester charges that she was a "murderer,"

> I thought I was going to go to Hell and God was going to punish me if abortion was murder—I was like 'Is abortion murder, maybe it is murder?' I just sat there and used to think about that constantly."

Providers were troubled when their patients internalized the idea that they were killers. One surgical assistant recalled a case in which a patient's nineteen-week dilation and evacuation was well underway when the patient began to cry and shout that the medical team was killing her baby:

> I'm just crying. . . . This procedure seemed to take forever, I'm sure it didn't. . . . So we walk out of the room and have to go right into seeing other patients . . . we're all like zombies. . . . It was a terrible, terrible feeling. I did try to contact her several times just so I could have some closure like for me, um, she never returned our calls, she never came back for her follow up.

Many workshop participants talked about fetuses, fetal parts, and their emotional responses to them. A counselor reflected on the difficulty she had the first time she looked at the remains of an aborted thirteen-week fetus:

At one point I thought to myself, I'm gonna have to look at some products [of conception] and [the doctor] said, "Oh, we've got a thirteen-weeker." . . . And she said she'd leave it out for me, so I went back into the surgery room, and there on a tray was a fetus, and I sort of was standing there with my hands behind my back sort of looking. . . . And I turned around [to the doctor] and said, "OK, I did it." And then I went back and finished my day and did a good job, but I thought, that was traumatic for me. . . . And does that mean I'm not cut out to do this work? I will lay down in front of a truck to protect a woman's right to choose, but that was really hard for me. So I was going back and forth, but I felt like, if I talk about that are people going to think you can't do this, you're not tough enough, you're not detached enough. . . . So I wonder if anyone else has ever sort of struggled about that.

The group members affirmed this participant's experience, sharing their own struggles and feelings. They also rejected the idea that an emotional reaction indicated unacceptable vulnerability or that staying detached was preferable. One physician asserted, "I am more guarded about not feeling. I never want to not feel." Another added,

As I always say, you can hold two things at the same time. But, just like with hospice . . . we get new people at hospice, and they say, "I'm crying all the time"—and I say, "When you stop crying, you need to find a new job." I mean you don't have to be crying in front of people, but when you're not feeling moved at some level about what's going on, then maybe you need to find a new line of work.

For these providers, struggling emotionally with aspects of the work wasn't troubling—it was how they knew they were still thoughtful and engaged with the work.

For some, these issues and feelings came into bold relief when watching fetal ultrasound images before an abortion procedure or while disposing of fetal remains afterward. One doctor shared,

We had someone pretty much deliver [her fetus before the procedure was underway]—and [the fetus] wasn't dismembered, the way all the other fetuses are. . . . We had this totally intact dead fetus. . . . Normally [it is]

in pieces we just put it in the bucket. But it felt so horribly wrong to just throw it in the bucket with all the fetal parts, so we got its own jar . . . and [the surgical assistant] went outside and picked some flowers and got some leaves, and we wrapped it up in one of the blue pads [as a blanket].

A medical assistant, reflecting on the second-trimester termination of a pregnancy complicated by a fetal anomaly, described watching a fetus on ultrasound as a doctor injected digoxin to stop the fetal heart before the procedure:

[The doctor] asks her . . . "Are you sure this is the right decision?" And she's like, "Yes." She starts to cry. "I can't—I have a kid that's two years old." And I'm like, all right, this is going to be a rough one. [The doctor] went to tell her, "You don't have to, this can be fixed," but that's not his job. His job is to do what she asked. And I wanted to say it at that point, but you know he's set up, he's doing his thing. Everything's going perfect, he inserts the laminaria. I'm fine; I've done [this] a million times. . . . He goes to do the dig[oxin], and puts his finger on her tummy, and . . . I'm watching it because I've never seen the ultrasound before. . . . And I see the fetus's hands start moving, and [the doctor] keeps poking this one spot, and the fetus like turns all the way around. And I'm like, "Ohhh, I don't know if I can do this." Like this fetus is saying, "Don't do this to me." My emotions start going haywire . . . and I look, and I see it. . . . I feel like I'm going to pass out or faint, and so I just look the other way. They finished. I pretend like nothing's wrong. I go about my day, and I go home, and I lost it. . . . And I had to question myself, like, can I do this? Because I really wanted to scream at that woman before that needle went in, "This is fixable! You don't have to do this!" But that's not my place. . . . I felt like woman taking care of woman, that was my job . . . putting the patient first before yourself sometimes.

This medical assistant's emotional response resonated with her co-workers. They offered support, not judgment, and emphasized their responsibility to the woman and her needs. One remarked,

This is such a heavy burden . . . and you don't have to feel it by yourself. I'm very clear that the fetus is not our patient, that the woman is. But sometimes . . . every once in a while, you still feel really sad. And that's OK. That's part of being a good human being.

The medical assistant agreed, saying she coped by telling herself to "always look at what [the patient] wants to do, [it's] not about anybody else . . . always put their feelings first, don't put anybody else's." Another added, "Many other people felt that way the first time they see dig[oxin]. It's human."

Tensions between Work Experience and Pro-choice Advocacy

The Expectation (and Burden) of Self-Censorship

Outside the workshop setting, abortion providers did not speak about the kind of experiences and feelings we have documented here. During the workshops, they not only shared stories but also reflected on their reasons for, and experiences of, silence. The providers maintained a habit of self-censorship for numerous reasons, including being looked down upon by advocates or endangering access to abortion. One physician remarked, "There's a real move amongst providers to euphemize, . . . if you say anything that embodies ambivalence or a kind of reflection and uncertainty you run the risk of restricting access and [appearing as if] you're not as committed to choice."

In a climate of restrictive legislation, calls to cut all public funding for reproductive health care at sites that also perform abortions, and several years marked by multiple undercover video sting operations attempting to implicate some abortion providers in illegal activity, the providers felt compelled to guard what they said. One provider recalled a stressful encounter with her sister:

> [She was] texting me all these questions . . . how many abortions do we do a day . . . who comes in for abortions, and how many boxes of Plan B we give out? All of the sudden instead of knowing that this is my sister, I was like, should I be answering these questions? . . . It's a very strange feeling to be suspicious towards a family member about work that you do. . . . And that's very much the politics of abortion. [I wondered] how the information would be presented and then maybe misconstrued, . . . because I wouldn't want any information that I give to construe [my organization] in a bad way at all.

Following that story, another provider remarked how cautious she's become—worried that her casual speech could be recorded and misappropriated:

> By capturing people saying things, perhaps out of context, . . . and then just posting it on YouTube . . . it makes it sound like we are evil and warped. . . . [Conversations] like when does life begin? Is it a baby or is it not? . . . All these things . . . we have to be cautious of. Are we really

pro-choice? Are we really giving information out in a way that is not tricking people into having abortions? You know, all the things that people accuse of us doing that we never do, yet any conversation [could be] taken out of context.

Self-censorship was an onerous burden. Although providers might like to share their work days with partners and friends, as people in other professions or other parts of medicine do, many do not feel able to. One physician stated, "I feel sometimes I'm held hostage by the work I've chosen to do because I can't be open about it." Another doctor sarcastically observed, "I had a really hard day at work today—I couldn't get the head out. Who can I tell that to?" She described sadness about losing connections that many other people enjoy. A clinic director echoed this sentiment of lost everyday connections: "It's the reality. It's the secrets that don't get talked about outside of here. . . . Can you sit at the dinner table and say, 'Oh, I felt horrible when I saw those fetal parts today'?" Many others spoke about these gaps in sharing their work lives with others. Said another, "I'm not going to talk about the jar [of fetal remains] outside of this building. . . . I don't know if I could explain this."

Questions of Language

Providers also reflected on differences between language used inside the clinic and accepted pro-choice rhetoric. Some noted that during clinical encounters they attempt to "meet their patients where they are" by using the words the patients use, such as baby instead of the more clinical term fetus. At the same time, clinicians' responses to other terms like "killing" were more complicated. As previously demonstrated, some providers opted to use this language, especially when reflecting a patient's own language. Others, however, rejected the word *killing*, finding it inconsistent with their feelings about the work or too reflective of antichoice rhetoric.

Providers expressed frustration with pro-choice rhetoric that did not align with their experiences in day-to-day work. Even though the workers themselves sometimes made similar distinctions, they felt that nonclinician advocates far too often emphasize stories about "worthy" abortions and "deserving" women likely to gain public sympathy (e.g., abortion in the setting of rape or fetal anomaly) to the exclusion of more common situations that lead women to choose abortion. As one provider put it,

For me, there's not [a] certain type; we see so many women from different ethnic backgrounds, financial background, religious, etc. . . . And everyone has a story of why they're here today. You hear some heartbreaking stories and then not so much heartbreaking. . . . There's just so many women that make this choice. And it's their body, it's their choice.

Some lamented the pro-choice movement's relative inability to use language to mobilize support, compared with that of the antiabortion movement:

> Speaking frankly is just something that the prolife movement does really well. . . . What kind of strong language do we have? You talk about women, but obviously it's not women who the prolife movement targets that they want to help . . . it's more babies—the children, the innocent, and women are not targeted as being innocent. . . . So being frank is really hard when you're talking about changing the political climate because you can't say we need to do abortion because abortions are a needed service; it's just not as easy.

Others expressed disappointment with the pro-choice movement's perpetual defensive stance, and with messages arguing for choice rather than for abortion. As one provider put it, "Why can't we have a pro-abortion stance?" Another wondered, "Can you say that on a bumper sticker?"

Lack of Connection to Movement Advocacy

For some providers, tension resulted from a perception that they were supposed to feel connected to movement advocacy and politics when they were not. "It's a paycheck," as one said. For others, the expectation to do the day-to-day work and be politically active felt like asking too much:

> It is really hard to stay connected to the political movement around women's health while working in the clinic because people will constantly ask you, "Oh, what happened around this?" and I'm like, "I don't really know," because you are kind of detached from that. You're working in the clinic, around women's health, but at the same time, because we have so few resources, you don't even have the time to do the work you're trying to do, the basic function of your job half the time, much less go the extra mile.

One participant actively avoided political news in order to manage the anxiety she felt that abortion would become illegal:

> My coping mechanism is what you said. I just don't read; I just don't give a shit. . . . I think it's like I will wake up one day and they will have overturned *Roe* and I will have to come up with another plan.

These tensions demonstrate the disaffection some providers feel with the politics surrounding abortion. Even so, many agreed that the movement is more vulnerable if its core workers lack political passion and engagement.

Experience of Sharing Silenced Stories

Even within the workshops, some participants worried that their stories would invite judgment from colleagues. However, most were quick to offer support, encouraged one another to be frank, and, in fact, connected this ability to share to a stronger abortion workforce. A counselor commented on the uniqueness of having a safe space for sharing stories as well as for addressing issues like burnout. "People are getting burnt out. . . . You know, we're not able to share, or I have to worry about if I share my feelings about something—I might be fired. [Here] we are able to share how we're feeling, or be angry, and not have to worry."

The providers said that the opportunity for sharing stories helped them feel revitalized and reconnected to their work. One counselor reflected, "Sometimes you kind of forget why you are here because every day you are just going with your routine. . . . It gave me a chance to go back and remember what my purpose was here." Many expressed a desire for more opportunities in the future. One observed, "This has been a pretty safe space to share and . . . at least release some of it, let a little bit go. It would be good to continue this in some kind of way." Another added that such opportunities "could be monumental for abortion care." Many emphasized the importance of sharing stories with the outside world to help generate greater support for abortion providers.

> I think this group has been very interesting because it really brings out a lot of emotions that you . . . shove . . . away—it doesn't even faze you anymore because you don't have that outlet to talk about it. . . . They [friends and family] have no idea what we go through, . . . and I think they need to; people need to know about that.

Discussion

Echoing the findings of other researchers, our data reveal the difficult aspects of abortion work, especially wrestling with views of abortion as killing, concerns (despite evidence against) about abortion causing fetal pain or causing patients pain, and the gruesomeness of dealing with fetal parts.[20] The providers acknowledged that they sometimes judge patients who fit antiabortion stereotypes or worry they fulfill these stereotypes themselves. Some admit to moral uncertainties. Furthermore, we note that abortion providers perceive that the pro-choice movement requires them to remain silent about the ethical and emotional complexities of their work. The providers worry that antiabortion advocates could use such disclosures to bolster claims that abortion is wrong and providers are cruel and uncaring. Therefore, providers do not speak openly about experiences that could pose a danger to the pro-choice movement.

We adopt the term *dangertalk* for these kinds of narratives and disclosures. Michelle Rosenthal introduced "danger talk" in her work in South Africa's first rape crisis center.[21] She found that Black clinic workers suppressed transgressive narratives about the intersections of race and gender. With the objective of promoting feminist empowerment for all women, the mostly White clinic leaders urged their members to avoid discussions of past and current racial injustices. They deliberately marginalized and sacrificed the experiences of some in the movement for the sake of unity of message.

In our work, we modify and expand upon Rosenthal's concept, using a compound word—dangertalk—to signal this elaboration. Rosenthal identified danger talk as a researcher and outside observer. We define dangertalk from the perspective of individuals within a movement who self-censor authentic experiences that feel dangerous to a movement they support and love. These individuals may also feel that the movement expects them to keep these dangerous experiences silent. We hypothesize that acknowledging dangertalk and reclaiming these marginalized narratives can be a powerful ingredient for revitalizing the abortion rights movement and social movements more broadly.

Is Dangertalk Dangerous?

At the heart of dangertalk is the assumption, shared by providers and advocates, that unedited sharing of providers' experiences is in fact dangerous for the pro-choice movement. Indeed, such disclosures could result in greater scrutiny from antiabortion forces and increased harassment. Some dangertalk narratives may reinforce antiabortion messages. Antiabortion advocates could use providers' words to validate their arguments and increase abortion stigma. Public discomfort with abortion procedures could also increase, leading to apathy or greater support for legal restrictions and reduced access. Dangertalk could make it harder to recruit and retain abortion workers by leading to increased stigma, violence, and burnout.

But might there be benefits? The workshop participants' narratives suggest that dangertalk performs several key functions that could strengthen the pro-choice movement. First, speaking about routinely censored topics provides a stress-release valve. Many providers in our study noted that the workshops left them feeling revitalized and better connected to their colleagues. Sharing these experiences in a supportive and reflective space helps to reduce the impact of stigma and its internalization among providers.[22] The participants spoke about the profound reassurance they experienced in learning that colleagues struggled with similar doubts and pressures.

Second, and importantly, the participants described their experiences with thoughtful, nuanced moral "sense-making" through exploring and voicing stories about their challenging work.[23] The group setting, in particular, provides an opportunity to connect through these stories, making dangertalk a touchstone for reducing rather than enhancing isolation by highlighting the similarities between workers' experiences and enhancing coping.[24]

Third, these psychologically complex depictions of providers can restore their humanity by unsettling the dichotomized stereotypes of providers as either heroes or butchers. Such depictions may help to normalize providers and the medical practice of abortion in the public's imagination. We expect this development could have a positive impact on abortion provider recruitment and retention efforts, and perhaps on the environment of hostility and distrust that currently surrounds abortion providers.

Fourth, interrogating dangertalk offers the pro-choice movement opportunities to grow, mature, and strengthen by developing new discursive messaging. Dangertalk reveals the ways providers talk about and manage their authentic, sometimes raw experiences, which typically only find a public home in anti-abortion rhetoric (e.g., harm to the fetus, inflicting pain, etc.). What would happen if, rather than shying away from the difficult, messy parts of abortion, the movement embraced them?

Dangertalk's Potential for Developing New Discursive Frames

Dangertalk highlights unspoken tensions within the pro-choice movement, perhaps particularly between providers and advocates. It offers new perspectives on abortion practice and therefore new opportunities for discursive framing and communication. As Carole Joffe and colleagues observed, although both providers and activists share a goal of keeping abortion legal and safe, there are points of contention, largely around issues of framing and discourse. Movement messaging emphasizes the importance of patient and woman-centeredness, largely delegating the provider to a technical role. Roe framed the exclusion of providers' experiences from movement messaging as a sign of the movement's immaturity.[25] Joffe and others have argued that for the movement to survive it is essential for health professionals and activists to align.[26] Creating a space for dangertalk—welcoming it, even—is an opportunity for such alignment.

All social movements produce collective action frames—carefully crafted strategic messaging to rally public support and attract new members to their causes.[27] Traditionally, abortion rights activists have framed messages from a feminist and patient-centered perspective which (rightfully) gives credence to women's point of view (e.g., "My body, my choice"). However, these same messages marginalize the experiences and expertise of providers. Historically, this would have meant marginalizing a largely male physician workforce seen by feminists as steeped in patriarchy. However, the contemporary abortion workforce is not only increasingly female but also younger and came of professional age in the setting of the women's rights movement.[28] They identify with these advocates and feel uncomfortable when at odds with their messages. Engaging with and understanding dangertalk may provide a way to enhance current discursive frames by adding back provider's voices.

As Nancy Naples argues, employing a materialist feminist analysis—one that explicitly acknowledges the dynamics of gender, race, culture, sexuality, and class—can "reveal how discourse and institutional practices organize the actualities of everyday life."[29] She posits that the process of creating message frames needs to include an interactional approach—one that is dialogic and dynamic and that positions a movement's organizational goals and strategies within larger institutional and political contexts. Dangertalk illuminates how cultural practices of the pro-choice movement silence the material, everyday experiences of abortion providers. Engaging in dangertalk expands a movement's capacity for holding complexity and self-critique.

The notion that dominant discourse marginalizes some members is not limited to abortion. Identifying and listening to marginalized voices is a common feminist analytic strategy within a range of social contexts. Therefore, we suggest that engaging in dangertalk in systematic ways could be useful in a variety of settings. Within intersectional feminist analyses, discussions of reproductive justice, trans rights, and feminism for women of color are just a few examples where one could likely find dangertalk narratives. We hypothesize that a formalized process for engaging in dangertalk could lead to more inclusive narratives within multiple movements.

Conceptual Model of Dangertalk

We present the following conceptual model, using abortion as a case study, in the hopes that others will find it useful to apply to their own fields of study. Our conceptual model illustrates a process for expanding abortion discourse through dangertalk (figure 9.1). The solid triangle represents contemporary dominant

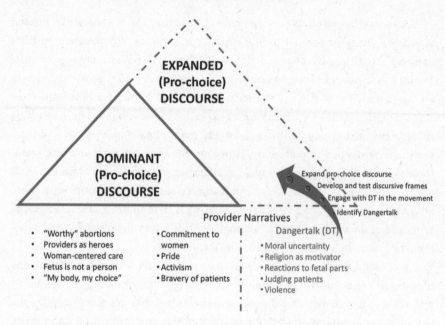

Figure 9.1 Conceptual model of dangertalk in U.S. pro-choice discourse

pro-choice discourse. Underneath this triangle we list examples of current messaging frames, including abortion care as a woman-centered enterprise: with choice as a central attribute and that a fetus is not a person and that abortion providers are heroes.

As the model depicts, some provider narratives align with the dominant discourse, including providers' commitment to caring for women, taking pride in their work, seeing their work as a form of feminist activism, and emphasizing the bravery of patients who move past protestors to get to the clinic (Harris et al., 2011). However, dangertalk narratives, which are currently outside the dominant discourse, focus on providers' moral uncertainty, stigmatization of religious values within the clinic, criticism of the pro-choice movement, negative emotional reactions to fetal parts, and judgmental attitudes toward patients.

The arrow illustrates that inviting these narratives into mainstream discourse could widen the tent, so to speak, of abortion messaging. The steps are to identify dangertalk narratives then to share these stories with insider groups. For us that includes other abortion providers and actors in the movement—such as activists, advocates, and communications experts. Next, craft new frames that include dangertalk themes and collaborate with experts on opinion research to test them. Finally, integrate these new tested message frames. We hypothesize that, taken together, these steps constitute a dynamic process in which social movements will mature and gain increasing comfort with nondominant narratives that come from within the movement. The enlarged discourse triangle will continually expand over multiple iterations.

How Dangertalk Could Reshape Abortion Discourse

The rise of state-level abortion restrictions in recent years demonstrates that abortion access is seriously threatened. The pro-choice movement must consider new strategies if abortion is to remain accessible for women.[30] At present, pro-choice and antiabortion discourses speak against and past each other. Liberating providers' stories offers rich material for building bridges across discursive divides.

For example, antiabortion rhetoric engages arguments founded on highly religious, largely Christian premises whereas pro-choice discourse typically relies on secular arguments. In our study, the participants described how their religious beliefs are congruent with choosing to provide abortions and how they view their work as an expression of their faith. Rather than yielding religious ground to antiabortion messages, the pro-choice movement can do more to articulate the ways in which religion plays a positive role in women's decision to have an abortion and providers' decision to work in this field. Better articulating this could perhaps foster empathy and identify shared purpose among those who find themselves on the opposite side of the abortion debate but are united in the centrality of religion in their lives.

Acknowledging the fetus, its meaning and value, may also make a powerful contribution to pro-choice discourse. As scholar/activist Francis Kissling has insisted, the pro-choice movement needs to rethink its exclusive focus on women while eclipsing entirely the significance of the fetus in the debates. Kissling argues "that people can hold contradictory things and complex values at the same time . . . and [the movement that] is able to talk both about fetuses and their value and about women is . . . going to win over the majority of the American people."[31] Similarly, Linda Layne astutely observed that it has been difficult for feminists to "acknowledge pregnancy losses without undermining women's right to end unwanted pregnancies."[32] Dangertalk stories that focus on the fetus reveal how meaningful these subjects are to providers and women they serve. The providers endow the fetus with great significance while prioritizing women's choices and interests. Avoiding these conversations can make the work feel more difficult for providers and contribute to stereotypes of providers as callous, unfeeling, and unaware of the nature of the work they perform.

Finally, what kind of radical shift might we see in the nation's polarization around abortion if some abortion providers routinely said, "Yes, abortion stops a beating heart, and sometimes I do think of my work as killing—and yet I find it the most fulfilling work I could do"? Our conversations could potentially shift away from purely descriptive ones—debates over what abortion is or is not—to ones based in meaning, motives, purpose. We see these developments giving rise to what David Snow and colleagues have called a "quotidian disruption"— one that challenges the "taken-for granted routines and attitudes of everyday life" and creates possibilities for activism.[33] We believe that this shift would contribute to a stronger pro-choice discourse, one that is less vulnerable to attacks based on semantic definitions of life and is increasingly informed by providers' moral conscience.

We anticipate that many people who otherwise support abortion will be uncomfortable with our findings and hypotheses. Indeed, this discussion itself is a form of dangertalk. Once published, the stories we report may (predictably) be appropriated by antiabortion groups for their own purposes. In fact, when we have presented these ideas at feminist conferences some have reacted with suspicion, worry, and concerns about "airing our dirty laundry." By contrast, in clinical family planning meetings we hear expressions of gratitude for our efforts to give voice to their experiences. Until new message scripts can be formally tested, it is clear that some will perceive these ideas as dangerous. However, to not share our work would reproduce the very self-censorship we critique and further efface and dishonor the experiences of abortion providers everywhere.

Conclusion

Abortion providers' current self-censorship practices—their avoidance of dangertalk—come with personal and social costs. It has allowed inaccurate and toxic representations of abortion providers and the women they serve to occupy the public sphere. These inaccurate representations in turn contribute to false pro-choice/prolife dichotomies, distorted depictions of women's lives, and a devitalized abortion rights movement. In order to restore what has been cut out of accounts of abortion provision, we argue that embracing dangertalk is essential. But engaging in dangertalk calls for the movement to create spaces for sharing and reflecting on the experiences and costs of censorship. This type of reflection and inclusion of dangertalk narratives could reinvigorate pro-choice discourse, where abortion is understood to be a human right and abortion providers are viewed as dedicated, compassionate professionals.

Abortion is but one context in which dangertalk can offer productive contributions. Dangertalk offers an approach for transgressive resistance where there is a gap between a group's rhetoric and the lived experiences of its members, resulting in censorship or self-censorship. Ultimately, we hypothesize that social movements, even social revolutions, are unfinished until they make room for dangertalk—until they engage dangertalk's potential to disrupt, complicate, and mature traditional discursive frames.

Notes

1. Carole Joffe, *Doctors of Conscience: The Struggle to Provide Abortion before and after Roe v. Wade* (Boston: Beacon Press, 1995); Carole Joffe, *Dispatches from the Abortion Wars: The Costs of Fanaticism to Doctors, Patients, and the Rest of Us* (Boston: Beacon Press, 2010); Wendy Simonds, *Abortion at Work* (New Brunswick, NJ: Rutgers University Press, 1996); Jeannie Ludlow, "The Things We Cannot Say: Witnessing the Trauma-tization of Abortion in the United States," *Women's Studies Quarterly* 36, no. 1–2 (2008): 28–41, http://dx.doi.org/10.1353/wsq.0.0057; Allyson Lipp, "Conceding and Concealing Judgment in Termination of Pregnancy; a Grounded Theory Study," *Journal of Research in Nursing* 15, no. 4 (2010): 365–378, https://doi.org/10.1177/1744987109347031; Lisa H. Harris, Michelle P. Debbink, Lisa A. Martin, and Jane A. Hassinger, "Dynamics of Stigma in Abortion Work: Findings from a Pilot Study of the Providers Share Workshop," *Social Science and Medicine* 73, no. 7 (2011): 1062–1070, https://doi.org/10.1016/j.socscimed.2011.07.004.
2. Simonds, *Abortion at Work.*
3. Kathleen M. Roe, "Private Troubles and Public Issues: Providing Abortion amid Competing Definitions," *Social Science and Medicine* 29, no. 10 (1989): 1191–1198, https://doi.org/10.1016/0277-9536(89)90362-6.
4. Allyson Lipp, "Stigma in Abortion Care: Application to a Grounded Theory Study," *Contemporary Nurse* 37, no. 2, (2011): 115–123, https://doi.org/10.5172/conu.2011.37.2.115.
5. Simonds, *Abortion at Work*; Roe, "Private Troubles"; Harris et al., "Dynamics of Stigma."
6. Anuradha Kumar, Leila Hessini, and Ellen M. H. Mitchell, "Conceptualising Abortion Stigma," *Culture, Health and Sexuality* 11, no. 6 (2009): 625–639, https://doi.org/10.1080/13691050902842741; Lipp, "Stigma in Abortion Care"; Harris et al., "Dynamics of Stigma."
7. Everett C. Hughes, "Studying the Nurse's Work," *American Journal of Nursing* 51, no. 5 (1951): 294–295; Carole Joffe, "What Abortion Counselors Want from Their Clients," *Social Problems* 26, no. 1 (1978): 112–121, https://doi.org/10.2307/800436; Harris et al., "Dynamics of Stigma"; Jenny O'Donnell, Tracy A. Weitz, and Lori R. Freedman, "Resistance and Vulnerability to Stigmatization in Abortion Work," *Social Science and Medicine* 73, no. 9 (2011): 1357–1364, https://doi.org/10.1016/j.socscimed.2011.08.019; Catherine Chiappetta-Swanson, "Dignity and Dirty Work: Nurses' Experiences in Managing Genetic Termination for Fetal Anomaly," *Qualitative Sociology* 28, no. 1 (2005): 93–116, https://doi.org/10.1007/s11133-005-2632-0.
8. Harris et al., "Dynamics of Stigma."
9. Harris et al., "Dynamics of Stigma."
10. Ludlow, "Things We Cannot Say."
11. Ludlow, "Things We Cannot Say."

12. Lisa H. Harris, "Second Trimester Abortion Provision: Breaking the Silence and Changing the Discourse," supplement 1, *Reproductive Health Matters* 16, no. 31 (2008): 74–81, https://doi.org/10.1016/s0968-8080(08)31396-2.

13. Lisa H. Harris, personal communication, 2009.

14. Simonds, *Abortion at Work*; Carole E. Joffe, Tracy A. Weitz, and C. L. Stacey, "Uneasy Allies: Pro-Choice Physicians, Feminist Health Activists and the Struggle for Abortion Rights," *Sociology of Health and Illness* 26, no. 6 (2004): 775–796, https://doi.org/10.1111/j.0141-9889.2004.00418.x; Harris, "Second Trimester Abortion Provision."

15. Lisa H. Harris, Lisa A. Martin, Michelle Debbink, and Jane Hassinger, "Physicians, Abortion Provision and the Legitimacy Paradox," *Contraception* 87, no. 1 (2013): 11–16, https://doi.org/10.1016/j.contraception.2012.08.031.

16. Paul Brink, "Heroes in Their Own Right: what Clinic Staff Do, and Why They Do it," Rewire News Group, June 24, 2015, https://rewire.news/article/2015/06/24/heroes-right-clinic-staff.

17. Roe, "Private Troubles."

18. Harris et al., "Dynamics of Stigma"; Lisa A. Martin, Michelle L. P. Debbink, Jane Hassinger, Emily Youatt, and Lisa H. Harris, "Abortion Providers, Stigma and Professional Quality of Life," *Contraception* 90, no. 6 (2014): 581–587, https://doi.org/10.1016/j.contraception.2014.07.011; Michelle L. P. Debbink, Jane A. Hassinger, Lisa A. Martin, Emma Maniere, Emily Youatt, and Lisa H. Harris, "Experiences with the Providers Share Workshop Method Abortion Worker Support and Research in Tandem," *Qualitative Health Research* 26, no. 13 (2016): 1823–1837, https://doi.org/10.1177/1049732316661166.

19. See Debbink et al., "Experiences with the Providers Share Workshop Method" for a detailed description of the methodology.

20. Susan J. Lee, Henry J. P. Ralston, Eleanor A. Drey, John C. Partridge, and Mark A. Rosen, "Fetal Pain: A Systematic Multidisciplinary Review of the Evidence," *JAMA* 294, no. 8 (2005): 947–954, https://doi.org/10.1001/jama.294.8.947; Simonds, *Abortion at Work*; Roe, "Private Troubles"; Ludlow, "Things We Cannot Say."

21. Michelle Rosenthal, "Danger Talk: Race and Feminist Empowerment in the New South Africa," in *Feminism and Antiracism: International Struggles for Justice*, ed. by Kathleen M. Blee and France W. Twine, 97–124 (New York: New York University Press, 2001).

22. Debbink, et al., "Experiences with the Providers Share Workshop Method"; Harris et al., "Dynamics of Stigma."

23. Kenneth J. Gergen, Mary Gergen, and Frank J. Barrett, "Dialogue: Life and Death of the Organization," in *The SAGE Handbook of Organizational Discourse*, ed. David Grant, Cynthia Hardy, Cliff Oswick, and Linda Putnam, 39–60 (Thousand Oaks, CA: SAGE 2004).

24. Debbink, et al., "Experiences with the Providers Share Workshop Method."

25. Roe, "Private Troubles."

26. Joffe et al., "Uneasy Allies."

27. David A. Snow and Robert D. Benford, "Master Frames and Cycles of Protest," in *Frontiers in Social Movement Theory*, ed. Aldon D. Morris and Carol McClurg Mueller, 133–155 (New Haven, CT: Yale University Press, 1992).

28. Emily Bazelon, "The New Abortion Providers," *New York Times*, July 14, 2010, https://www.nytimes.com/2010/07/18/magazine/18abortion-t.html.

29. Nancy A. Naples, "'It's Not Fair!' Discursive Politics, Social Justice and Feminist Praxis SWS Feminist Lecture," *Gender and Society* 27, no. 2 (2013): 133–157, https://doi.org/10.1177/0891243212472390.

30. "Last Five Years Account for More Than One-quarter of All Abortion Restrictions Enacted since Roe," Guttmacher Institute, January 13, 2016, https://www.guttmacher.org /article/2016/01/last-five-years-account-more-one-quarter-all-abortion-restrictions -enacted-roe.

31. Francis Kissling, "Op-Ed: Time for a New Approach to Abortion Rights," *NPR*, February 21, 2011, https://www.npr.org/2011/02/21/133941176/Op-Ed-Time-For-A-New -Approach-To-Abortion-Rights.

32. Linda L. Layne, "Unhappy Endings: A Feminist Reappraisal of the Women's Health Movement from the Vantage of Pregnancy Loss," *Social Science and Medicine* 56, no. 9 (2003): 1881–1891, https://doi.org/10.1016/s0277-9536(02)00211-3.

33. David Snow, Daniel Cress, Liam Downey, and Andrew Jones, "Disrupting the 'Quotidian': Reconceptualizing the Relationship Between Breakdown and the Emergence of Collective Action," *Mobilization: An International Quarterly* 3, no. 1 (1998): 1–22, https://doi.org/10.17813/maiq.3.1.n41nv8m267572r30.

Part 4

The Fetus

Over the past two centuries, the status and image of the fetus has changed significantly. Once considered objects belonging to pregnancy and family, fetuses attracted scientific attention in the nineteenth century when physicians began to attend miscarriages. Hoping to learn more about pregnancy and the fetus, physicians sought access to fetal specimens and presented miscarried fetuses for study at professional meetings. The first essay in this section by Shannon Withycombe discusses the ways in which the new medical interest in fetuses contributed to the redefinition of the fetus from family object to object of scientific study and set in motion a process that led to important discoveries about pregnancy and fetal bodies. Eventually, it prompted the development of technologies and treatments used today in neonatal intensive care units (NICUs) to keep fetuses healthier and premature infants alive at earlier gestational stages.

By the turn of the twentieth century, physicians began to use tissue from aborted fetuses and nonviable fetuses—fetuses that might still show signs of life but were too immature to survive outside the womb—for medical research. Neuroanatomist Davenport Hooker was one of the earliest and most influential researchers to use nonviable fetuses. Anthropologist Lynn Morgan described how, between 1932 and 1958, Hooker performed neurological tests on 149 fetuses at the University of Pittsburgh. Local doctors notified Hooker when they expected a premature delivery or planned a therapeutic abortion. Hooker would retrieve the fetuses and bring them to his laboratory where he immersed them in a saline solution warmed to 90 degrees Fahrenheit to perform neurological tests during the brief period—between seven and twenty minutes—when the fetuses were still alive. He recorded the neurological responses on motion picture film, footage of which he assembled in 1952 into an educational film called *Early Fetal Human Activity*.[1] Many other researchers used nonviable but still living fetuses for research into the 1960s. They did so in a cultural context in which fetuses did not carry the same meaning they do in the early twenty-first century. As Morgan noted, "It is not that Hooker, his colleagues, or his audience de-humanized the fetus or hardened themselves against its charms. They had no charming fetuses in their repertoire; they had never humanized fetuses to begin with."[2]

In the 1960s, popular writers began to disseminate the scientific findings, and images of fetuses appeared in general publications. Several of Hooker's images, for instance, were published in 1962 in an early pregnancy guidebook by Geraldine Lux Flanagan, *The First Nine Months of Life*.[3] Three years later, *Life* magazine published a photo essay by Swedish photographer Lennart Nilsson entitled the "Drama of Life Before Birth" which revealed for the first time what a developing fetus looks like. Nilsson obtained the images from women who terminated their pregnancies under the liberal Swedish law. Working with dead embryos allowed Nilsson to experiment with lighting, background, and positions.[4] The dissemination of these images helped to transform public understanding of the fetus, and the general public began to regard encounters with the dead fetus as distasteful and macabre. This change in the understanding of the fetus also undermined the conditions that had allowed for the research and creation of the images in the first place. After the 1960s, researchers rarely publicized the fact that fetal images came from dead or dying specimens.[5]

Prior to the legalization of abortion, fetal research evoked little public concern. Investigators quietly planned, funded, completed, and published fetal research without drawing public attention. Fetal research in the 1960s and 1970s involved the fetus inside and outside the uterus and addressed a wide range of questions: knowledge of normal fetal growth and development, fetal disease or abnormality, fetal pharmacology, and the effects of chemicals and other agents on the fetus to develop fetal therapies and techniques to save the lives of premature infants. Research on dying fetuses and on tissue cultured from fetal cells led to important discoveries, such as our knowledge about fetal development and the 1954 development of the polio vaccine. By 1969, tissue from an infected aborted fetus from the Washington Laboratory allowed investigators to develop a rubella vaccine, thereby protecting future generations of mothers from miscarriages or stillbirths and infants of infected mothers from severe birth defects. Other researchers used fetal tissue to develop tests for Rh incompatibility to avoid complications in pregnancy as well as birth defects and amniocentesis screenings to detect other genetic anomalies. The most extensive and invasive procedures included attempts to keep the fetus alive and led to the development of technologies and therapies that today are part of NICUs and have, over the years, pushed fetal viability earlier and earlier.[6] If, in the early 1970s, the point of fetal viability was generally twenty-eight weeks after conception, a decade later it was possible to sustain the lives of infants as early as twenty-three weeks.[7]

The legalization of abortion politicized fetuses. Antiabortion activists recognized that putting a spotlight on fetal research could serve their broader political strategies and goals. Tapping into larger discussions about the protection of human subjects, opponents of abortion treated the fetus as a vulnerable subject, suggesting that a fetus was no different from an infant. Legal abortion, they argued, was a convenient avenue for physicians to gain access to research subjects.[8] To provoke emotional and protective responses toward the fetus, antiabortion activists placed images and descriptions of fetuses and fetal suffering at the center of their strategy. Physicians who performed abortions and scientists who engaged in fetal research, they implied, held no consideration for fetal life and acted with deliberate disregard when they performed abortion procedures. By the mid-1970s, the modern views of the fetus clashed with older scientific sensibilities.

The biological, legal, and ethical differences between an early fetus wholly dependent on the pregnant woman and the more developed fetus that might survive outside the womb became particularly sensitive. To guide debates surrounding fetal research, a group of bioethicists discussed the status of the fetus, whether or not it was considered a person, and whether or not it was entitled to rights and protections. The fetus, advocates of fetal research argued, was not a person but an "object" that had value only insofar as it was wanted by its parents. Only once it became a live-born baby, capable of independent existence, did it acquire personhood.[9] Philosopher Richard Wasserstrom concluded that research on a nonviable fetus scheduled for abortion with no potential to develop into a human being was permissible if it would yield information otherwise unobtainable. And philosopher and ethicist Sissela Bok argued that research experiments on viable fetuses were permissible if the research sought to benefit the fetuses used as subjects or their families, if researchers sought to develop new techniques for helping premature infants survive, or if they sought to test new diagnostic techniques that could not be tested at an earlier gestational age.[10] And many medical researchers praised the accomplishments of fetal research, pointing to advances in fetal therapeutics that had resulted from research on the fetus.[11]

But another group of ethicists strongly argued that ethical standards governing fetal research should be the same as those governing research on children or other vulnerable subjects. Because abortion was immoral, Richard A. McCormick concluded, investigators should only conduct research on a fetus for which abortion was not contemplated.[12] Many denounced research on the fetus as dehumanizing and feared its implications for society. A professor of neurology at George Washington University sarcastically demanded that the fetus be protected from experimentation "without its informed consent."[13] Others expressed the fear that research on the fetus might persuade women to have an abortion in order to contribute to the cause of science.[14]

Opponents built their case against fetal research by focusing on research to develop life-support systems for fetuses and on studies of fetal metabolism. This research involved fetuses that were alive but not viable, and hence was aesthetically most disturbing. Abortion opponents described fetal experiments in graphic terms, creating a narrative in which fetal specimens were really fragile infants who were subjected to horrendous medical experiments while still alive. In the process, abortion opponents intentionally distorted and trivialized scientists' research goals, claiming for instance that researchers seeking to understand the impact that complications from maternal diabetes might have on fetal development were merely trying to solve frivolous dietary questions about coffee sweeteners.[15]

While the bioethics discourse addressed significant moral dilemmas, it failed to resolve many of the issues. Bioethicists frequently emerged with lists of guidelines and recommendations that might offer physicians a blueprint on how to act. But these resolutions did not constitute a consensus. A second essay in this section, "A Feminist Defense of Fetal Tissue Research" by Thomas Cunningham, explores contemporary arguments for and against fetal research.

Fetal research also led to the emergence of neonatology as a specialty and NICUs as the place to care for premature infants. The term neonatology first appeared in a 1960 text *Diseases of the Newborn*.[16] Between the 1960s and the 1980s, neonatology grew, and by 1982 there were 600 neonatal intensive care units with 7,500 beds. Born prematurely, NICU patients suffered from immature lungs, frequently accompanied by cardiac, neurological, and gastrointestinal problems. The smallest of these infants died within hours of their birth. In the 1960s, pediatricians aggressively treated premature infants with new technologies developed at the borderline between fetal research and the emerging new subspecialty of neonatology. By the 1970s, improvements in neonatal care meant that the infant death rate in the first month of life was almost cut in half. In 1960 only 10 percent of infants born at 1,000 grams (2.2 pounds) survived, but a decade later half of the infants survived.

As physicians developed therapies and technologies to keep younger and younger infants alive, they confronted both the promises and limits of neonatology. Over the course of the decade, physicians came to realize that outcomes for many infants were poor. Survivors of NICUs, a 1973 article in the *New England Journal of Medicine* pointed out, were at times severely handicapped by a myriad of congenital malformations that in previous times would have resulted in early death.[17] "Yesterday's heroic efforts are today's routine procedures," one pediatric surgeon described the situation as he questioned the utility of the new therapies.

> Each year it becomes possible to remove yet another type of malformation from the "unsalvageable" category. All pediatric surgeons, including myself, have "triumphs"—infants who, if they had been born 25 or even five years ago, would not have been salvageable. Now with our team approaches, staged surgical technics [*sic*], monitoring capabilities, ventilatory support systems and intravenous hyperalimentation and elemental diets, we can wind up with "viable" children three and four years old well below the third percentile in height and weight, propped up on a pillow, marginally tolerating an oral diet of sugar and amino acids and looking forward to another operation.[18]

Maybe, the surgeon implied, it was time to think more critically about the long-term outcomes premature infants might face rather than focus on viability over all other factors.

Parents, too, were concerned about aggressive medical interventions that seemed to have no good outcomes. Other considerations than the mere preservation of life, they suggested, should be part of clinical decision making. The quality of life of the infant, the cost of medical care, and the emotional burden on remaining family members all played a role in parental considerations. In the 1960s and early 1970s, a series of cases in which parents refused to give permission for a simple life-saving surgery because their infant suffered from Down's syndrome drew attention to the issues of parental autonomy and decision making in the NICU. Throughout the 1970s and early 1980s, cases such as these caught the imagination of the general public and raised the question whether parents should have the authority to forgo medical care for infants born with a disability.

By the mid-1970s, conference participants from medicine, law, theology, philosophy, and the social sciences pondered the question whether it was morally legitimate for physicians to forgo life support for compromised infants. While they tended to affirm that parents had the right to make such decisions, the attendees also agreed that it was desirable to save the lives of infants who may be "marked by physical and intellectual abnormalities."[19] The question of when to sustain the life of premature or seriously compromised infants thrust neonatal care into the ambit of the early bioethics movement and prompted vociferous debate.

By the early 1980s, the election of President Ronald Reagan and the rise of the religious right had politized fetal and infant life. In 1982, a six-day-old infant known only as Baby Doe died at Bloomington Hospital in Indiana after his parents, with approval of the courts, denied him food, water, and surgical aid, and the case led to a national outcry. Born with Down's syndrome, Baby Doe also suffered from a condition in which the esophagus is not connected to the stomach, which is correctable with surgery. Commentators across the country condemned the parents for letting their infant starve to death, the infant's physicians for ceding to the parents' wishes, and the courts for refusing to step in. Outrage echoed all the way to Washington, DC, where, a month after the death of Baby Doe, the Reagan administration issued a "Notice to Healthcare Providers" informing hospitals that they ran the risk of losing federal funding if they withheld treatment or nourishment from "handicapped" infants.[20] The final essay, by John Colin Partridge, illuminates the ways in which neonatologists have assessed the conditions of NICU patients, deliberated on when to elect comfort care and when to provide more aggressive interventions, and sought to develop indicators that would aid their decision making about the treatment of their patients.

Notes

1. Lynn Morgan, *Icons of Life: A Cultural History of Human Embryos* (Berkeley: University of California Press, 2009), 197–199. Hooker tried to slow down asphyxia and fetal death but was unsuccessful.
2. Morgan, *Icons of Life*, 201. Morgan notes that Hooker and other researchers like him avoided criticism by maintaining a high standard of professionalism and integrity. Hooker was well connected professionally and was known as a conscientious researcher. His publications focused strictly on the scientific merits of the project, and he was always careful to mention that the fetuses in his study came from operations "undertaken only after the most careful consideration and after extensive consultation" (*Icons of Life*, 201). Hooker also stressed that no member of his research team was ever involved in a decision about whether to perform a therapeutic abortion.
3. Geraldine Lux Flanagan, *The First Nine Months of Life* (New York: Simon & Schuster, 1962).
4. Albert Rosenfeld and Lennart Nilsson, "Drama of Life before Birth," *Life* 58, no. 17 (April 30, 1965): 54–72A.
5. Indeed, as Morgan points out, Hooker's research was appropriated in support of pro-life causes. Antiabortion activists cited Hooker's work to make the point that "babies" are "responsive to touch" (Morgan, *Icons of Life*, 204–205). And by the 1980s, antiabortion activists had embraced the aesthetic display of fetal bodies and begun to disseminate images of dead fetuses and fetal remains.

6. National Commission for the Protection of Human Subjects of Biomedical and Behavioral Research, *Report and Recommendations: Research on the Fetus*, Publication No. (OS) 76-127, vol. 1 (Bethesda, MD: U.S. Department of Health, Education, and Welfare, 1975), 14–15.

7. Dena Kleiman, "When Abortion Becomes Birth," *New York Times*, February 15, 1984, https://www.nytimes.com/1984/02/15/nyregion/when-abortion-becomes-birth-a-dilemma-of-medical-ethics-shaken-by-new-advances.html, 14.

8. Melva Weber, "Middlemen in the Definition of Life," *Medical World News*, November 22, 1974, 61. For a brief history of fetal research, see Sara Dubow, *Ourselves Unborn: A History of the Fetus in Modern America* (New York: Oxford University Press, 2011).

9. National Commission, *Report and Recommendations*, 32.

10. National Commission for the Protection of Human Subjects of Biomedical and Behavioral Research, *Appendix: Research on the Fetus*, Publication No. (OS) 76–127, vol. 2 (Bethesda, MD: U.S. Department of Health, Education, and Welfare, 1975), 2–15.

11. National Commission, *Appendix*, 44.

12. National Commission, *Appendix*, 34–35; also 31–39.

13. National Commission, *Appendix*, 45.

14. National Commission, *Appendix*, 45.

15. *Congressional Record*, H3428, April 25, 1974, as quoted in David W. Fisher, "Editorial: A Rampage of Know-Nothingism," *Hospital Practice* (June 1974), file: Abortion Update 1974, series Abortion, Takey Crist Papers, Sally Bingham Center for Women's History and Culture, Duke University Libraries, Durham, NC.

16. Alexander J. Schaffer, *Diseases of the Newborn: With a Section on Neonatal Cardiology* (Philadelphia: Saunders, 1960).

17. Raymond D. Duff and A.G.M. Campbell, "Moral and Ethical Dilemmas in the Special Care Nursery," *New England Journal of Medicine* 289, no. 17 (1973): 890–894, https://doi.org/10.1056/nejm197310252891705, here 890.

18. Anthony Shaw, "Dilemmas of 'Informed Consent' in Children," *New England Journal of Medicine* 289, no. 17 (1973): 885–890, https://doi.org/10.1056/nejm197310252891704, here 889.

19. A. R. Jonsen, R. H. Phibbs, W. H. Tooley, and M. G. Garland, "Critical Issues in Newborn Intensive Care: A Conference Report and Policy Proposal," *Pediatrics* 55, no. 6 (1975): 756–768, https://doi.org/10.1542/peds.55.6.756, here 756.

20. Norman Fost, "Putting Hospitals on Notice," *Hastings Center Report* (August 1982): 5–8, https://doi.org/10.2307/3560759.

Chapter 10

How Science Is Made

Nineteenth-Century Embryology and Fetal Interpretations

Shannon K. Withycombe

Current debates about reproductive rights and justice often hinge upon physiological and anatomical fetal developments: when can the fetus feel pain? When is there a detectible heartbeat? What structures does a ten-week fetus share with a full-term infant? Right-wing conservatives use scientific findings (the appropriateness of calling their arguments "scientific" is the topic for another article) as proof that abortion is equal to murder. What no one on either side of these political debates recognizes is how we, as a culture, came to know these scientific "facts."

The development of a fetus into a fully formed child takes place within the hidden world of the uterus. There is no window to the inside, and even in the twenty-first century, technologies for long-term or repeated viewing of development carry risks. Instead, most of what we know about embryological development comes from embryos and fetuses that exited the mother's body in some fashion—abortion, miscarriage, and removal during hysterectomies or other surgical procedures. The emergence of modern American embryology in the early twentieth century depended on an older tradition of physicians removing miscarriage products—dead, alive, or in between—from the intimate space of the bedside of a miscarrying woman.[1]

In 1866, Mr. B, a young man in Crestline, Ohio, visited Dr. J. Stolz to ask the physician for help. Mr. B's wife was in much pain and distress, and he feared for her life. Stolz accompanied the young man back to his house where he found the sixteen-year-old woman thrashing about in bed, screaming in pain. After an examination, Stolz determined that the woman was having a miscarriage and that "labor had proceeded so far, that its arrest was impossible." An hour later the woman delivered a five-month-old fetus. The doctor wrapped the fetus in a flannel and laid it aside on a sofa, turning back to his patient who was bleeding considerably. After "giving the usual remedies" to the mother (probably a morphine derivative or ergot to promote uterine contractions to expel the placenta), Stolz turned back to the fetus and was surprised to find it still alive, "gasping for breath, [and] making regular inspiratory movements." Stolz took the fetus with him when he left the house, and as he reported later in a medical journal, "I carried it to my office, where it was also witnessed by my professional friends, Drs. Booth and Jenners. It gradually succumbed, after surviving its birth one hour and forty minutes. It measured about six inches in length."[2]

Numerous physicians removed miscarriage products (embryos, fetuses, and placentas) from the homes of miscarrying women in the second half of the nineteenth century. Like Stolz, they frequently shared them with colleagues, sometimes with large audiences at medical society meetings or through the pages of medical journals. Miscarriage products ended up in doctors' offices, medical school classrooms, and museums all across the country. So customary was the practice of securing miscarried embryos and fetuses in American medicine that by the early 1900s, when Franklin P. Mall, an eminent embryologist at Johns Hopkins University, decided to build a collection of human embryological specimens, he was able to gather thousands of "creatures" (as many physicians called them) in only a few short years. Over 500 physicians helped Mall, passing along their treasures for what became the largest clearinghouse of embryological knowledge in the nation. Doctors' common practice of acquiring miscarriage remains enabled the creation of a collection that was used to establish the modern stages of fetal development.

Nineteenth-century physicians, all over the country and coming from a variety of backgrounds, seemed united in their interest in what miscarriage products could help teach them. While they may have individually differed on what important information fetal and placental tissues could provide—the causes of miscarriage, the process of fetal development, the mechanisms of conception, or even the very meanings of life and death—male physicians agreed that these "creatures" were highly valuable for the progress and professionalization of scientific medicine. By investigating the social and scientific constructions of meaning for fetal and embryonic tissues in the nineteenth century, we can better understand our current evaluation of such materials as scientific samples, political tools, and markers of family tragedy.

Tiny Bodies

In March 1839, Dr. A. Lopez was summoned to attend "Louisa, a coloured woman," or more specifically to attend to what had come out of her uterus. Two days earlier, Louisa had delivered a healthy child with a midwife in attendance. The women caring for her decided to call in Dr. Lopez to help decipher a newly discovered object: a small body "which had been thrust aside unobserved, on the day of parturition, among the soiled clothing and discharges."

Intrigued by the object, Lopez took the fetus away from Louisa's bedside and house and placed it in a bottle of alcohol for preservation. He then attempted to transport the specimen from South Carolina to Alabama in order to present his treasure before the Medical Society of Mobile. Along the way the bottle broke, the alcohol evaporated, and the entire surface of the fetus became covered with mold. Then, while attempting to clean the specimen, Lopez inadvertently detached the umbilical cord, effectively ruining an important aspect of the specimen: the coiling of the cord around one knee and thigh. In May 1845, Lopez presented the object before the Medical Society of Mobile, Alabama. Even in its moldy and damaged state, the small body became the topic of a lengthy discussion at the meeting and, ultimately, a twenty-two-page article on a variety of subjects, including the necessity of female orgasm for successful conception, the origin and preserving powers of amniotic fluid, and the possibility of spontaneous amputation within the womb.[3]

Let us consider many important aspects of this case. As a member of an elite medical society in the South, Lopez was undoubtedly White. Louisa, a "coloured woman" in South Carolina in 1845, was probably enslaved. The power dynamic between patient and practitioner would have constructed a situation where Lopez would not have needed to consider Louisa's cooperation before absconding with her bodily discharges. In addition, Lopez probably construed Louisa's body as many White southern physicians did in antebellum America as being stronger, more animalistic, and impervious to pain or modesty by virtue of her race. Nineteenth-century physicians, almost exclusively White elite males, discussed Black women, particularly under slavery, as lacking in the capacity for sentimental motherly affection, care, or bonds. Within this framework, Lopez would not have thought twice about taking Louisa's miscarriage products away, regardless of whether she felt empowered enough to say anything.

We do not know how Louisa did or would have interpreted her miscarriage products, but we do know that once in the hands of Dr. Lopez, those materials became a "specimen." By virtue of her race and social position, Louisa was robbed of the opportunity to interpret what came out of her body and what to do with it. To be sure, it was not merely at the bedside of a miscarrying woman that White society stripped Black women of their mothering. Taking Louisa's four-month fetus away from her would have made sense to an elite White society used to seeing enslaved Black women separated from their children, even infants. But Lopez's reconstruction of Louisa's fetus into a specimen also mirrored concurrent medical use of Black bodies in antebellum America. Scholars have long addressed the racial construction of anatomy writ large in nineteenth-century medical development. Medical schools all over the country utilized bodies of disenfranchised groups, often to get around cadaver laws, in their studies of anatomy and physiology. A Black fetus in a jar would have fit right into American medical science of the time.[4]

It was not only the racial dynamics in antebellum and Jim Crow America that enabled the growth of embryological science but also the growing reproductive restrictions that led to changing views of miscarriages. Unless a family deemed the fetus to be of little personal value, doctors could in many cases not remove the fetus from a family's home, be it alive or dead. As one physician bemoaned after delivering a set of twins he estimated to be between four and five months' gestation, "I made an earnest effort to secure the children . . . to preserve as specimens, but failed, the parents objecting to it."[5] Among White families, then, women had agency in these decisions, and they, their families, and their female attendants played an important role in decisions about miscarriage products.

In the second half of the nineteenth century, many American couples became newly interested in limiting their family size. This was especially true among the growing urban working poor who had limited physical space for families, or among the expanding middle class who increasingly viewed fewer children as a sign of status. However, at the same time, state and federal governments criminalized abortion and birth control, leaving most Americans with unreliable, costly, or nonexistent fertility control measures. In such circumstances, some women found comfort in having a miscarriage and considered the products more akin to a specimen than a child. For most of the cases reported in medical journals, late nineteenth and early twentieth century, families did not view miscarriage products as "children" or "babies," but as rather something of which to dispose.

In January 1875, Annie Van Ness miscarried her first pregnancy; unlike most modern miscarriage narratives we see on blogs or in pregnancy advice manuals, she wrote of the event as a joyous occasion. Van Ness was twenty-seven at the time and just over a year into her married life. More importantly, her husband Theodore had lost all his money in the Panic of 1873, just before their marriage. The couple had been forced to relocate and adopt a new way of life that included strict budgeting. This might have been why, upon realizing she was pregnant, Annie Van Ness wrote in her diary, "I am very cross and irritable and I think I have very good reason to feel ill humored." Two weeks later, Van Ness miscarried and described her mood: "I am happy again."

Van Ness did not describe what came out of her body as a child, something to mourn, or a valued family member. Instead she wrote, "it wasn't any larger than a jointed doll." Van Ness saw something with a humanistic (or at least doll-like) body, but rather than grieving the loss of an infant, she described herself as "pretty smart" after the event. As a young wife juggling her new economically strained life, Van Ness may not have been ready for the cost and responsibility of an infant. And living in a state in which abortion and birth control were outlawed, Van Ness may have resented her lack of control over her own fertility. In this context, miscarriage did not evoke grief or create a dead child, but instead evoked relief and created something of more use to a physician than to a family.[6] Since the miscarriage went smoothly and Van Ness's mother helped her through it, there seemed no reason to call a doctor. But if she had, there is every reason to imagine she would have happily handed over the resulting tissues as a medical specimen.

It is within this context that we can better understand the social reactions to miscarried fetuses, even ones which held little physical differences from a full-term infant. In 1852, Dr. A. W. Barrows presented a case before the Hartford Medical Association. Barrows had attended Mrs. J, a woman who in the article seems to bear all the signs of being White and respected. Barrows had visited Mrs. J during her fifth month of pregnancy and helped her deliver a fetus completely encased in its sac. To Barrows's surprise and amazement, the fetus was still alive. Upon rupture of the membranes, the fetus uttered a cry, it breathed for forty minutes, it stuck its tongue out at various intervals, it made occasional voluntary movements of the extremities, and its heart beat for three-quarters of an hour. Viewing this case as one of extraordinary value in how it proved viability in a fetus so young, Barrows made careful observations, recording every structure and function he saw, including hair, fingernails, arterial pulsation, skin color, pupils, muscle development, and head shape. This tiny female body, measuring ten inches in length and weighing fourteen ounces, provided a unique view into embryological development usually unobservable to medical practitioners.[7]

Barrows's specimen was deemed so valuable by the medical society to which he presented it that they voted on its great value to the medical profession and sent the report on to a national medical journal. But this great medical and embryological specimen was only available for study because neither Barrows nor Mrs. J and her family treated the fetus as a child. Barrows kept watch over the fetus, as he says, "with interest and care," but did not describe any attempts to aid with respiration, keep it warm, or offer any other life-saving techniques for premature births common at the time. The scientific knowledge gained by Dr. Barrows and his colleagues was dependent on the dehumanization of the fetus by all those involved, physicians and family alike.

The Proper Place

By the close of the nineteenth century, multiple physicians had presented human fetuses at medical meetings, discussed them at length in medical journals, displayed them in museums, and used them in their teaching practices, all without any public censure. But this did not mean that Americans viewed the fetus as an object lacking value. Instead, by looking at scandals involving the discovery of fetuses in public spaces, we can see the success physicians had in reformulating the fetus into a scientific specimen.

Popular narratives described the public disposal of fetal tissues as barbaric. A woman's bedroom or a scientific setting had, by the late nineteenth century, emerged as the only two proper places for a fetus. Barrows and other physicians did not simply remove fetal and embryonic tissues, sometimes alive, from homes and families. They made a concerted effort to recast these tissues into scientific specimens, perhaps aware that if they did not reshape a human fetus into a scientific object, they faced severe public disapproval and could lose the much-needed support of the families who involved them in miscarriage cases.

In 1898, Joanna R. Nicholls Kyle wrote a story for the popular publication *Godey's Magazine* after a visit to the Army Medical Library and Museum in Washington, DC. In what would turn out to be the last year of the long-running and popular women's magazine (previously known as *Godey's Lady's Book*), Kyle described visiting the new public museum, which housed thousands of human specimens. The Army Medical Museum got its start during the Civil War, when then U.S. Surgeon General William Hammond directed all Union doctors to collect examples of injuries and disease and ship them to his office for cataloguing and future study. The collection quickly grew: body parts, organs, skin sections, and photographs of a wide variety of bodily ailments. By the 1880s, the collection, now including any human specimen deemed worthy of study, was so large the government was forced to construct a new building for the books and specimens, which was completed in 1887.

Kyle visited the museum in 1898 and filed a detailed report on the history of the museum, its current collection, and its role as a tourist attraction. According to Kyle, the collection held over 33,000 specimens, including gunshot wounds, a wide variety of bones, skin diseases, sections of frozen bodies, drawings of parasites, wax models of sperm and egg, and a large series of human fetuses and embryos in jars. Keeping her popular audience in mind, Kyle reported on particular objects of interest, such as "a bit of human skin on which an arrow had been tattooed." The fetuses on display there, framed within glass and mounted in a scientific manner, garnered no outrage or criticism, but instead they seemed to Kyle to fit perfectly within the larger world of research and science.[8] In its' first decade, tens of thousands of tourists visited the Army Medical Museum each year to see the array of specimens. And perhaps most, like Kyle, viewed the embryological display with wonder and excitement. While describing the examples of skin conditions as "revolting" and the displays of the ravages of diseases as "hideous," Kyle used the term "delicate" when discussing the fetuses in jars. At the end of the article, Kyle promoted the museum as valuable to the public for entertainment and education, in particular an excellent venue for class trips or outings for families with young children.

In contrast to Kyle's article, a *New York Times* article from 1877 brings us the story of Mrs. Mary Tait and her miscarriage. Mrs. Tait was rushed to the New York Hospital after receiving two stab wounds in her abdomen. Five days later she delivered a six-month-old fetus and returned home soon after. The hospital morgue received a burial permit for the fetus and sent Dan Russel, the driver of the dead wagon, to collect the fetus. When Russel arrived, "he was told by the clerk that he guessed the body had been thrown into the furnace and cremated. Dan's astonishment and horror at the supposed barbarity of the physicians knew no bounds." When a *Times* reporter interviewed physicians at the hospital, one stated that he did not understand the protests and actually "seemed greatly amused at the interest created by the occurrence." Another stated that if the fetus had been cremated "he could see nothing improper in it. He did not know whether such a proceeding was common in hospitals, but it was common to burn parts of limbs that had been amputated." It was, after all, the doctor reported, the most effective method of disposing of them.[9] Located neither in a bedroom nor a lecture hall but rather in a hospital furnace, a location typically reserved for amputated body parts or other waste, this fetus was in a liminal space between child and specimen, between person and depersonalized body.

Other newspapers described the discovery of fetuses in public spaces, found distinctly outside of science, as criminal if not abhorrent. In 1895, two boys fishing in the Missouri River in Sioux City, Iowa, discovered a human fetus floating along wrapped in a bed quilt.[10] In 1898, a human fetus was discovered in the hills around Los Angeles.[11] In both cases, police quickly became involved; even though the authorities could not determine how the fetuses arrived in the river or the hills, each case was depicted as a deplorable crime. When a fetus became separated from either familial or scientific realms, as with these cases, words such as "barbarity" were bandied about.

Looking beyond medical journals for discussions of the fetus as science reveals how successful physicians were in reshaping the fetus into a specimen. The transformation of miscarriage products into fetal specimens became an accepted image of the fetus in public spaces. In magazines and newspapers of the late nineteenth century, nonscientists viewed the fetus as properly belonging to either the family or science.

Conclusion

Remarkably, while physicians did not interpret the products of miscarriage as infants, they still saw them as clear representations of humans, thus enabling embryological research that helped construct the modern pregnancy as one that primarily focuses on a developing infant. Anatomical and physiological developments that personalize the fetus, such as when the heart starts to beat—a milestone favored by antichoice groups and obstetricians alike as "proof" of the child—entered twentieth-century pregnancy advice and obstetrical practice only after families and doctors categorized miscarriage products as specimens rather than people. Now, as contemporary reproductive rhetoric relies on the embryological "facts" presented in medical texts, ultrasound images, and public health propaganda, it conveniently erases its own cultural history of how this supposedly "objective" knowledge came to be in the first place. Our ability to know when fetal heartbeats start, or when hair grows, or when a fetus can feel pain depends directly on women and their doctors first agreeing on the quasi-human status of miscarried fetuses.

In 1849, Dr. Charles Munde assisted his own wife through a miscarriage at five months, ending his report: "After twenty-two hours from the beginning of the accident, the foetus, a boy (whom I preserve in alcohol) went off."[12] This scenario—a doctor delivering what many would consider today his own son, yet putting the fetus in a jar of alcohol for preservation—seems foreign and strange. But these historical accounts remind us that miscarriage, like all health and bodily conditions, is socially constructed. Munde lived in a society in which doctors readily gathered up fetal specimens from miscarriage cases and studied them, preserved them, shared them, and learned from them. Munde also lived in a society in which families struggled to limit the number of children they had, at times welcomed miscarriage, and faced no reprobation for allowing a physician to leave their home with a (sometimes living) five-month-old fetus.

That is not the society we live in today, but it is dangerous to think that miscarriage is now somehow imbued with certain inalienable meanings as a death, a tragedy, and wrong. Millions of women still face struggles with obtaining safe, reliable, and affordable means to control their fertility, and certainly some of them welcome miscarriage as a result. Forcing families to categorize miscarriage as the death of a child, as numerous states have attempted to legislate in the past decade, only harms families and women. Even for those who do think of their miscarriages as a tragedy, unnecessary laws governing fetal remains cause undue burdens on families in terms of cost and physical and mental harm.

As many nineteenth-century women and physicians understood, grieving a miscarriage does not necessarily involve losing a person. It can, of course, but it can also embody a wide range of meanings: losing an opportunity, an idea, a fear, or a source of anxiety. In order to truly support families, we must not impose a universal meaning or moral judgment on an event that means different things to different people in different circumstances.

Notes

1. An earlier version of this essay appeared as "Meaning and Materials of Miscarriage: How Babies in Jars Shaped Modern Pregnancy," on the *Nursing Clio* blog, October 31, 2018.
2. J. Stolz, "Repsiration and Signs of Life in a Five Months Foetus," *Medical and Surgical Reporter* 15, no. 16 (1866): 344–345.
3. A. Lopez, "Account of a Blighted Foetus of the Third Month, Having the Umbilicus Cord Extensively Coiled around the Right Knee and Lower Third of Thigh, Discharged with a Living Child at Full Term," *American Journal of the Medical Sciences* 24 (October 1846): 309–330.
4. For further reading on the use of African American bodies in the development of American medical science in the nineteenth century, see Deirdre Cooper Owens, *Medical Bondage: Race, Gender, and the Origins of American Gynecology* (Athens: University of Georgia Press, 2017); and Stephen Kenny, "How Black Slaves Were Routinely Sold as 'Specimens' to Ambitious White Doctors," *The Conversation*, June 11, 2015, https://theconversation.com/how-black-slaves-were-routinely-sold-as-speci mens-to-ambitious-white-doctors-43074.
5. T. R. Rubush, "Superfoetation," *Transactions of the Indiana State Medical Society* 43 (1892): 181–187.
6. Annie L. Youman Van Ness, *Diary of Annie L. Van Ness, 1864–1881* (Alexandria, VA: Alexander Street Press, 2004).
7. A. W. Barrows, "Case of Abortion, Occurring at the Fifth Month of Gestation—Child Born Alive," *American Journal of the Medical Sciences* 50 (April 1855): 308–384.
8. Joanna R. Nichols Kyle, "The Army Medical Library and Museum," *Godey's Magazine* 136 (April 1898): 408–418.
9. "Cremation in a Hospital: A Dissected Fetus Burned in a Furnace," *New York Times*, August 26, 1877, 12.
10. "Boys Find a Fetus," *Sioux City Journal*, 1895.
11. "Another Mystery," *Los Angeles Times*, December 10, 1898, 11.
12. Charles Munde, "Water in Miscarriage," *Water-Cure Journal* 9, no. 6 (1850): 190–191.

Chapter 11

A Feminist Defense of Fetal Tissue Research

Thomas V. Cunningham

Introduction

In 2015, a prominent bioethicist responded publicly to a pro-life group's attacks on Planned Parenthood, which have been a regular occurrence in American politics. In the *New England Journal of Medicine*, Alta Charo noted that the political move made by that group was to portray Planned Parenthood as trafficking in human body parts, and particularly the body parts of the most vulnerable humans: human fetuses. Against this, she suggests we should all remember that every one of us has benefited from fetal tissue research: "Every child who's been spared the risks and misery of chickenpox, rubella, or polio can thank the Nobel Prize recipients and other scientists who used such tissue in research yielding the vaccines that protect us (and give even the un-vaccinated the benefit of herd immunity)."[1] But, as Charo notes, a response to this counter awaits: "Critics point to the underlying abortions, assert that they are evil, and argue that society ought not implicitly endorse them or even indirectly benefit from them, lest it encourage more abortion or make society complicit with what they view as an immoral act."[2]

In this way, Charo reveals how the battle lines are drawn on the issue of the morality of fetal tissue research. There are those who believe there is a standing moral imperative to perform research on human embryonic and fetal tissue precisely because of the special status of those tissues: what little we know about embryonic and fetal tissues suggests they are capable of a level of plasticity unlike other germline or somatic tissue and could yield biotechnological advancement. But just as there are those who believe that it is morally permissible to perform research on these tissues, others believe fetal tissue research is immoral because it harms the most vulnerable of human beings. Indeed, the U.S. Department of Health and Human Services changed federal policy in June 2019 to restrict funding for research using fetal tissue by requiring approval of an Ethics Advisory Board before funding such research. Yet since 1975 Republican administrations have effectively prevented controversial research on embryonic cells and fetal tissue by refusing to charter the very board necessary to approve the funding for research.[3] The justification given by the Department of Health and Human Services for this also follows directly from a paradigmatic "sanctity of life" position that such research is necessarily immoral because of the harms it will cause vulnerable human beings at the very beginning of life: "Promoting the dignity of human life from conception to natural death is one of the very top priorities of President Trump's administration."[4]

Although the debates about the legality and ethical permissibility of abortion care are long-standing, with the advent of in vitro fertilization, cloning, regenerative medicine, and other biotechnologies these debates have been exported into related, but distinct, social deliberations.[5] I aim to set aside the larger debate concerning the morality of abortion care and instead focus on the topic of the morality of fetal tissue research. While the two themes are connected, my approach will be to hold them at arm's length, where possible, for the purpose of conceptual analysis, with the goal of questioning whether progress may be made on the topic of the morality of fetal tissue research when it is distinguished from the morality of abortion care.

Ethics, Metaphysics, and Policy

In "Begging the Question: Fetal Tissue Research, the Protection of Human Subjects, and the Banality of Evil," Thomas Babbo argues that our current federal policies regarding fetal tissue research are immoral. His argument begins by noting that the Nuremberg Code prioritizes voluntary, autonomous choice:

> The most influential of the Nuremberg Code's conditions . . . was the necessity of obtaining authentic, uncoerced informed consent from human subjects. All codes and regulations to follow concerning the rights of human research subjects, both ethical and regulatory, would import this notion of informed consent with varying degrees of strictness and success.[6]

Babbo then spends a significant amount of time justifying the second part of this claim, that future regulations import the notion of informed consent found in the Nuremberg Code. Babbo shows how Nuremberg's emphasis on autonomous, voluntary choice runs through 1966 U.S. National Institutes of Health

(NIH) guidelines for protection of human subjects, the 1975 National Commission report on fetal tissue, and the 1979 Belmont Report.[7] His citation of the National Commission Report exemplifies this analysis:

> Throughout the deliberations of the Commission, the belief has been affirmed that *the fetus as a human subject* is deserving of care and respect. . . . [T]he members of the Commission are convinced that moral concern should extend to all who share genetic human heritage, and that the fetus, regardless of life prospects, should be treated respectfully and with dignity.[8]

Things changed, according to Babbo, in the early 1980s when the U.S. Department of Health and Human Services implemented new regulations of human subjects research, known as 45 C.F.R. § 46 or the Common Rule. In his view, the new regulations and resulting language of the 1993 Statute on Fetal Tissue Transplantation Research in the National Institutes of Health Revitalization Act caused a shift from protecting human subjects because of their inherent humanity and dignity to protecting human subjects when doing so is justified by "an 'end-justifies-the-means' utilitarianism."[9]

Given Babbo's dialectic, it is important to briefly consider the Common Rule regulations in some detail. The Common Rule governs all scientific research, including defining the purview and aims of institutional review boards, the mandate for informed consent for human subjects research, and the requirement of protection of vulnerable subjects. The regulations state that investigators have an obligation to obtain informed consent from a subject or that subject's legally authorized representative. The revised 2018 version of Common Rule expands upon what it means to procure such consent, including requiring that the language an investigator uses to procure consent must be "information that a reasonable person would want to have in order to make an informed decision."[10] The regulations also define groups of vulnerable persons and types of tissue that require special protections, including pregnant women, children, human fetuses, neonates, the placenta, the dead fetus, and fetal material.

Of particular importance for this analysis is how the regulations constrain procurement of fetal tissue from abortions:

(h) No inducements, monetary or otherwise, will be offered to terminate a pregnancy;

(i) Individuals engaged in the research will have no part in any decisions as to the timing, method, or procedures used to terminate a pregnancy; and

(j) Individuals engaged in the research will have no part in determining the viability of a neonate.[11]

Also, it is important to highlight the special mention of the placenta, the dead fetus, and fetal material:

(a) Research involving, after delivery, the placenta; the dead fetus; macerated fetal material; or cells, tissue, or organs excised from a dead fetus, shall be conducted only in accord with any applicable federal, state, or local laws and regulations regarding such activities.[12]

Babbo argues that the Common Rule rightfully draws attention to vulnerable populations deserving of special protections but while doing so it "introduce[s] a discordant view of humanity into the regulations: that a specific *class of human beings*, unwanted aborted fetuses, are not worthy of the same respect as other human beings."[13] Thus, what makes funding and performing fetal tissue research immoral, per Babbo, is that it both entails a commitment to a flawed consequentialist (e.g., utilitarian) reasoning *and* that it requires an ontological distinction between "aborted fetuses" and other human beings—a distinction Babbo clearly presumes spurious.

In prior work, I have taken on this ontological distinction directly in the case of embryonic tissues, where there is a standing presumption that, all things being equal, all embryos have the potential to develop into human beings and thus warrant the attribution of moral status consistent with their metaphysical status.[14] I have rebutted this view in the case of human embryos when compared to clone embryos. I will not re-cover that ground here except to say that if a competent clone embryo can be shown to be ontologically (and thus morally) distinct from a human embryo, then it would seem even more evident that a deceased fetus with no potentiality would be ontologically (and thus morally) distinct from a human being. I believe a different rejoinder to Babbo and those who would find him compelling may be crafted by invoking arguments developed within analytic feminism.

Relational Autonomy and Fetal Tissue Research

One response to Babbo's view is to point out that aborted fetuses are not alive and thus they do not fall under the regulations of human subjects research in the requisite sense for his argument to go through. That is, begging a crucial question regarding whether an aborted fetus is a human being in a morally meaningful sense of the term, Babbo seems to hold that previously living human beings—now-deceased human fetuses—ought to be regulated in just the same way as living human beings (perhaps like neonates or children). One might argue, however, that this is absurd in a basic sense: at most, tissue harvest from a deceased fetus (fetal tissue) is morally similar to tissue harvested from a deceased human being, as opposed to morally similar to a living human being of any age. Yet no doubt Babbo would demur, saying,

> In the context of donating fetal tissue . . . *the mother* of an unwanted, aborted fetus does not share the same status as a family member under [federal regulations]. By acting to end the life of her fetus, *the mother* has essentially renounced her maternal interest with respect to the fetus, and consequently has not the standing to provide surrogate consent for the fetus for the purpose of organ donation. Furthermore, state common law and statutory views of the standard of care required from a surrogate decision maker require the surrogate to consider the best interests of the patient.[15]

At this point, shouting might ensue, and then retrenchment. One could challenge Babbo's presumptive use of the term *mother* in this quote; without the birth of a living child, some previously pregnant women would reject attribution of this status and the social stigmas it invokes unto them.[16] Or one might concede that, of course, prior to their abortion fetuses are alive in a meaningful sense (yet one might not concede this either).[17] Regardless, one could still argue that a woman's liberty rights override a state's right to intervene to protect the potential life of the fetus, which would be to rehash decades of contentious legal precedent and philosophical argument.[18] We've been there. We may never leave.

I want to take a different tack. I aim to develop a response to a Babbo-esque argument against funding and performing fetal tissue research from an explicitly feminist stance. I see two distinct yet related ways to do this. First, it is possible to problematize the entire framework upon which Babbo's account rests. We may question what it means to see respect for autonomy as a foundational ethical principle, which Babbo rightly attributes to Nuremberg and later regulations. Second, we may question what it means to carve out special protections for vulnerable persons in our laws and to what extent such protections are based on gendered conceptions of normality that are biased against women.[19]

One of the earliest explicitly feminist contributions to bioethics scholarship comes in the form of a critique of the central notion of respect for autonomy. The decades following the publication of Jennifer Nedelsky's article, "Reconceiving Autonomy: Sources, Thoughts and Possibilities," have seen further development of the idea that the hallowed concept of *autonomy* that was dominant in early academic bioethics is so deeply flawed as to warrant revision.[20]

In sum, scholars in feminist bioethics claim that classical notions of *autonomy* are overly individualistic: they explicitly or implicitly assume a model of persons that abstracts them from their sociocultural contexts. In response, scholars have developed an alternative account of autonomy, *relational autonomy*, which refers to a conception of the self and its relation to the world that specifically recognizes one's embodiment and embeddedness in a social and cultural context. According to this view, a person's identity should be understood as being situated in their social environment, including their interactions with others and their own experience of being an embodied person with a lived identity. On this view, "the fact of interdependence pervades this relational understanding of the self, as people are only dependent and independent relative to the circumstances in which they find themselves."[21]

Quite simply, relational autonomy emphasizes *relationships*. So, in order to establish a being's rights and responsibilities, one is directed to consider its relationships to others. In those relationships, one will find the meaning of that being's existence, which provides context for decisions the being makes or others make on its behalf.[22] In the case of fetal tissue research, it is very difficult to see how *fetal tissue*—as opposed to *the fetus*—is capable of participating in meaningful relationships with other persons that are noninstrumental. Granting the very controversial premise that a fetus warrants equivalent moral status to all other human beings, after abortion a fetus becomes "fetal tissue." At that time, the tissue is no longer capable (in any sense of the term "capacity") of developing the ability to relate to other human beings. It thus seems quite simple that fetal tissue cannot be the bearer of (relational) autonomy.

We can imagine how an emphasis on relational autonomy would undermine Babbo-esque defenses of a view of humanity where fetal tissue is accorded the same ontological and moral status as fetuses, neonates, children, adolescents, and adults. Of course, this is to take the easy way out, Babbo will respond. He will call attention to *how* a fetus becomes fetal tissue and underscore that someone has to authorize an abortion in order for this to happen and then someone has to perform an abortion. He will point to the moral culpability of the first act and then gesture at how it "taints" all subsequent acts.[23]

Again, we've all seen this movie before. Perhaps there is no way out of it. But relational autonomy at least seems to change the terms of the debate. On the relational autonomy paradigm, recall that the patient is a self-governing whole, who is embodied in a particular place and time, with a particular personal, social, and cultural history. To adopt relational autonomy suggests that while a woman may have any number of relationships with fetal tissue, fetal tissue lacks the necessary capacities to have relationships with a woman. There is an asymmetry in the capacities of agency and self-governance that an individual woman has and fetal tissue does not. In her *self*-governance, she both cannot reject this embodiment and is entitled to reimagine it for the purpose of making her own choices. If the concept of relational autonomy were to become more widespread and were to displace more individualistic notions of autonomy, then it may, thus, provide a means to both undercut attempts to imbue fetal tissue with moral status and further emphasize a woman's right to make autonomous (medical) decisions about her tissue, fetal and otherwise.

Protecting the Pregnable (Someone Has to Help Them!)

Relational autonomy is well known in feminist circles and bioethics, to such an extent that it has been canonized in the only authoritative text in the field, Beauchamp and Childress' *Principles of Bioethics*.[24] Yet I find the discussion above an inadequate response to Babbo-style arguments. The major weakness appears to be that the concept of relational autonomy, despite its radical veneer, is quite consistent with the dominant paradigm of voluntary consent—only now with more attention to the person consenting and her sociocultural context. This emphasis on autonomy is precisely what Babbo appeals to in his arguments against fetal tissue research. Thus, even though relational autonomy draws attention to the humanity and autonomy of all women, especially those making medical choices, and reinforces the view that fetal tissues (and perhaps fetuses) lack the prerequisites for autonomy, it still seems an insufficiently radical response to Babbo's claims.

I see another way to defend funding and performing fetal tissue research drawing on feminist theory. Much has been made in bioethics and research ethics about the Common Rule's emphasis on vulnerable persons. On its face, it no doubt appears progressive to provide added protection for specific groups under the law; however, the specific groups singled out for protection, the language used to define those protections, and the practices of implementing these regulations have unexpected implications, which, once acknowledged, provide additional resources for rejecting Babbo's conclusions.

As mentioned previously, the Common Rule singles out pregnant women, children, human fetuses, and neonates as groups of vulnerable persons. It also singles out prisoners. I will focus on how singling out pregnant women as a category of vulnerable persons has affected research on a group of people who Vanessa Merton characterizes astutely with the phrase "pregnant, pregnable, and once-pregnable people (a.k.a. women)."[25] I want to then suggest that heeding calls for reform of these regulations and for countermeasures to alter the current research trends could impact fetal tissue research by empowering women to elect to donate fetal tissue.

As Merton and others have documented, until the early 1990s biomedical research was disproportionately performed with White male subjects. In her now-classic argument, Merton describes the many ways in which women have been disproportionately prevented access to participation in biomedical research and the disproportionately negative outcomes they bear as a consequence. Merton shows that women have been prevented from participating as human subjects due to explicit exclusion criteria in research protocols and they also have been inadvertently prevented from participation in research because researchers have failed to recruit them or have implemented research protocols that are biased in ways that make it more difficult for women to participate than for men.[26] The most important ill effects of women's lack of access to participation in biomedical research are that we know less about women's illnesses, we know far less about how therapies approved by the U.S. Food and Drug Administration affect them and the children they bear if they choose to do so, and there are fewer therapies for illnesses that specifically affect women (and children) or that affect women in ways that differ significantly from (White) men. Merton and others have covered this story in great depth, including that progress is being made on the issue.[27] According to Anne Drapkin Lyerly and colleagues, "women now make up the majority of participants in clinical research," yet disparities in research on women's health and the effects of therapies on women (and children) persist.[28]

In her article "The Perils of Protection, Vulnerability and Women in Clinical Research," Toby Schonfeld investigates how conceptualizing all pregnable (and once-pregnable) people as vulnerable has affected their statuses as persons and potential research subjects.[29] Because, as she notes, the Common Rule does not define "vulnerability" except to suggest it means being more likely to be "vulnerable to coercion or undue influence," Schonfeld draws on work by other scholars to provide a taxonomy of "vulnerability" and then proceeds to show, bit by bit, what it means to classify women as vulnerable. These categories of vulnerability include *cognitive, juridic, deferential, medical, allocational, infrastructural*, and *social* vulnerability. I focus on her analysis of only two of these categories.

Schonfeld defines juridic vulnerability as vulnerability that obtains when someone has legal authority over the decision making of another person. For example, parents have legal authority to make decisions for children, prison officials have legal authority to make decisions for prisoners, and military officers have legal authority to command enlisted soldiers to act.[30] Schonfeld points out that it could be reasonable to interpret this as applying to fetuses and pregnant women, but she notes that this legal notion fails to capture much that is meaningful about the relationship between a pregnant woman and a fetus. She further shows that the language of the Common Rule extends similar protections to the fetus as those extended to children.

> The implication with fetuses, therefore, is that all research involving the potential for direct benefit to the fetus alone must be considered to be of a sufficient risk to require what is known as "two parent consent." Yet recall that the fetus exists dependently with the woman, so that any risk to the fetus *is also a risk to the woman.* . . . The implication of conferring juridic authority on the father, then, is that it gives him the power to consent for research that will happen to someone *who does not lack decisional authority.* This is odd, to say the least. The regulations remain silent on what happens if the mother and the father disagree . . . although presumably refusal by one would fail to meet the criteria that consent is obtained by both parties. Regardless, the purported juridic vulnerability of the fetus has the paradoxical effect of making the pregnant woman juridically vulnerable, which gives others authority over choices affecting her own body—a situation we would judge unethical in any other population retaining cognitive decisional capacity. Therefore, as it stands, the regulations do not protect the rights and welfare of pregnant women who are research participants; rather, *they serve to create additional vulnerability for the pregnant women.*[31]

Schonfeld comes to a similar conclusion when examining the category of social vulnerability. In her account, social vulnerability is the most common type of vulnerability to which pregnant women are subject. This can be seen in terms of societal norms that women conform to expectations, such as limiting their consumption of alcohol or caffeine while pregnant. Schonfeld observes these same types of norms occurring in the context of research, where they take the form "of an attitude of protectionism towards the fetus. The regulations make it clear that risk to the fetus is the operative concern, and therefore, that all decisions—and decision makers—should focus on ways to minimize risk to the fetus, sometimes at great cost to the pregnant woman herself."[32]

In Schonfeld's scholarship, we find an argument for the conclusion that rather than *protect* women, categorizing all pregnant, pregnable, and once-pregnable people as vulnerable and requiring extra protection in human research for them has had the paradoxical effect of *making women more vulnerable.* The regulations express a systematic conceptual bias toward a vision of women, qua their status as potential childbearers, as unable to make moral choices about fetal health and thus as warranting "protection"—or in other words, undue influence and coercion to force them to attend to their potentiality as persons who can gestate and birth children. And, as other scholars have shown, the downstream effects of these biases have been to expose women to increased risk, to reduce our knowledge of women's bodies and illnesses, to limit how informed women's choices may be even when they are empowered to make them, and to limit their inclusion in biomedical research that might reduce risk and increase knowledge.

What should we make of this? My modest proposal is that by listening to insightful voices like Schonfeld's we may question the meaning of "protection," even when it is well meaning, look more carefully at our regulations, and call for reform. Attending to analytic feminist analyses in some detail suggests that revisions to national policy warrant reform in order to better protect women's liberty interests. More attention to such analyses and their implications by policy makers and the scholars whose work they consult may aid in building a better world for women, where they are more empowered to make more informed choices and freer from institutional, societal, and regulatory constraints.

In addition, Schonfeld's argument can be brought to bear on Babbo-style attempts to prohibit fetal tissue research. Both feminist approaches I have sketched out lead to the same end: they each aim to further empower women to make choices about their medical care and the method of disposing fetal remains.[33] Drawing on feminist theory allows us to question the assumptions of the dominant paradigms that infuse our regulations and structure the conceptual, political, and sociocultural environments in which we make choices as long as the ability to make choices remains protected and respected. As a response to Babbo, these arguments permit us to agree with him in a way. We can encourage his reformist intuitions. But then we, too, can point out the implications of language and concepts of humanity entailed by the regulations. And we can say that women and girls should be seen as human, all too human, just like boys and men. To do this is to draw attention to the humanity of women and require equal conceptualization of them in the regulations and equal treatment of them in practice. And, by focusing attention on women and their capacity and right to make choices, we may thereby draw attention away from the fetus and the putative moral status of fetal tissue without having to be drawn into unending metaphysical debates.

What Do Women Want?

While there thus seems to be a promising feminist defense of fetal tissue research, I also foresee an important limitation to this approach that is worth
mentioning as a counter to the optimism expressed earlier. One of the bedrock
principles of feminism is that, via various modes of oppression, women have
been denied their basic liberties and that working toward more respect for—
and ultimately fully securing and protecting—these liberties is a basic good.[34]
Analytic feminists have argued that an important route for performing this work
is to analyze concepts such as truth, rationality, and justice, and that in doing
so to justify assertions about existing constraints on women's freedoms and ways
to overcome them. This way of conceptualizing feminism assumes that there is
something common to women as a group that makes it possible to analyze a
shared circumstance and to delimit methods for improving that circumstance,
which has been called the assumption of the *univocality of "women."*[35] My
worry is that the same values that underlie this assumption could be drawn on
to support restrictions on fetal tissue research. Specifically, I worry that it is possible that a plurality of women in a given locale could move to constrain other
women's freedoms in the same region precisely because the exercise of their
freedoms engenders justified democratic constraints on the freedoms of others.
They may view their beliefs about restricting fetal tissue donation and research
as legitimate constraints to other women's countervailing beliefs.

To explain this worry, I will appeal to a nascent field of research on British
women's views about donating fetal and embryonic tissues to scientific research.
Owing to the Abortion Act of 1967 and the Polkinghorne Guidelines of 1989,
women have been able to donate fetal tissue for research in Great Britain for
decades.[36] Recently, British scholars have begun to examine the implications of
this practice, specifically with regards to informed consent for scientific research;
the meaning of the concept *fetus* implied by these practices; and the views of
men and women involved with donating tissues, with reproductive medicine,
or with research using fetal or embryonic tissues.[37] This research has been performed in very small British populations and thus serves as a poor basis for making inferences about even *most* women in *some* contexts, but its conclusions
are nevertheless informative.

The earliest research into British women's views about donating fetal tissue for research was motivated by the authors' recognition of the fact that while
the Polkinghorne Guidelines for fetal tissue research took many viewpoints and
perspectives into account, "no attempt was made to seek the opinions of women
of reproductive age, and in particular of women about to have a termination of

pregnancy."[38] To fill this gap, the authors surveyed 167 women who requested terminating a pregnancy but had not yet, 108 women with a history of terminating a pregnancy, and 419 women with no history of abortion about their views of fetal tissue research. The researchers found that the surveyed women overwhelmingly supported the idea of donating fetal tissue for research. They reported that 94 percent of them "felt that [fetal tissue] research was justifiable" and that more than 84 percent of the women surveyed thought that research into the basic physiology of fetal development was appropriate and that they would allow such research to be performed on their own fetus. The researchers found little variation of significance between the three surveyed groups, which is at least partially explained by the high levels of support for fetal tissue research among them.

In response to the 1994 survey, a more recent study used a focus group methodology to explore what matters to British women who are asked to think about donating fetal tissue for research. The focus groups included forty-one women, thirty-one of whom had previously had an abortion. The results of the study provide a sharp contrast to the earlier survey results. Women in this study reported feeling a prolonged attachment to fetal tissue when contemplating the prospects of its continued use by an abstract scientific researcher.[39] The focus group participants were initially supportive of the idea that fetal tissue could be used to better understand fetal development, but they changed their views about the prospects of donating fetal tissue the more they discussed its possible uses in research. For example, one participant noted, "You don't think of a fetus as just a bunch of human cells because, you know, it's embedded in your knowledge and your culture as to what a fetus can become."[40] Another participant said she was concerned that "if I agreed to have this fetus in medical research, I'd be thinking, what are they doing with it, you know? . . . I would really want to know, then it would bring more emotional side effects."[41] Discussing her findings, Pfeffer concluded, "In all of the focus groups, we observed a clear pattern where participants changed their position on the core questions of the rights and wrongs of donating a fetus for stem cell research as they gained information and thought more carefully about the implications of the decision."[42]

Comparing these two studies suggests a way in which the sort of feminist defenses of fetal tissue research described above might be undermined. The key difference in the two studies is that the survey study developed its inquiries in response to national guidelines, whereas the focus group study used facilitating methods to bring participants' beliefs and opinions about fetal tissue research to light without drawing the participants' attention to particular aspects of the topic of discussion. In this sense, the survey study can be seen as a top-down approach to asking women about their values and preferences relating to fetal tissue donation and research, while the focus group study is a bottom-up approach. Consequently, the focus group approach simulates personal relationships more so than the survey method: The participating women had a lengthy (guided) conversation in small groups while enjoying a bit of red wine. And in this context, they learned from each other about their different presumptions regarding fetal tissue research and the morality of donating fetal tissue. This education included vague statements, half-truths, personal experience, and all of the other hallmarks of communication between thoughtful, reflective peers. It is interesting that in this environment the women moved from a position of support for donating fetal tissue to one that combined apparent tolerance with disapproval. While it was not clear that the focus group participants would prevent others from donating fetal tissue, it was clear that they no longer approved of the prospect of donating fetal tissues resulting from their own pregnancies and abortions at the time the focus group concluded.

The survey and focus group studies come to very different conclusions about what women want in the context of fetal tissue research. The survey suggests most women believe fetal tissue research is either morally permissible or morally obligated, and that they endorse it. The focus groups suggest that women find the prospects of fetal tissue research morally troubling and that they disapprove of it while being disposed to tolerate others' choices to engage in it.

No other published, empirical research on the specific issue of British women's values and preferences toward fetal tissue research exists to clarify whether one of these assessments is more accurate than the other.

Yet work on the related issue of views on experimentation with embryos suggests that potential donors of embryonic and fetal tissues are more likely to have complex, diverse views about donation of, and research with, these tissues than the 1994 results from Fionn Andersen and colleagues would indicate.[43] Again, however, the research was extremely limited, amounting to only one focus group and interview study of fifty women and men in Scotland who were members of fertility support groups and undertaking the process of assisted reproduction. In this study, the participants expressed misconceptions about stem cell research that might follow from the donation of embryonic tissues. Most believed that donated embryos would only be the "spare embryos" that were unacceptable for use in fertility treatments because of physiologic abnormality. The participants also expressed an assumption that the "spare" embryos would be used for research within the field of reproductive medicine. They expressed a felt obligation to participate in such research, which is captured by one woman's quote: "Other people have given up for the research for us to get to this point so I feel as though well why shouldn't I do something for couples coming along?"[44] But this feeling was contextualized by the view that this obligation does not extend to research outside of reproductive medicine, as one man voiced: "I would like these embryos to go to treating infertility or helping people treat infertility. Not for any other purposes, because that was the reason that we came in the first place."[45]

In this small sample of individuals participating in fertility support groups, we see a similar attitude to those engaging in open discussion about the prospects of donating fetal tissue: people are worried about the beliefs and practices of scientists, they feel that donation and research might be appropriate for the purposes of improving the lot of others who might be in their circumstances one day, and they feel moral concern about using these tissues in research, especially if that research extends beyond reproductive science and medicine.

While the three studies here are extremely limited in their evidential value because of lack of replication and the narrow populations they were performed in, they do provide limited support for the intuition that women (and men) may have divergent views on the permissibility of embryonic or fetal tissue donation and research. This should not be surprising given the pluralism of British society. It is likely the same results would be found with larger studies in other settings. Let us take on the assumption, then, that women are pluralistic in their values and preferences regarding fetal tissue donation and research. My concern is that if *most* women came to feel this way in a particular locale, then they might move to legislate protections of fetal (or embryonic) tissues in line with their values. In this way, it is possible for such a group to be acting consistently with the basic principles of analytic feminism and yet still to lobby for, secure, and implement legal restrictions on other women's abilities to participate in scientific research by donating fetal tissues or by performing that research.

In some sense, this line of argument could be run on any issue, given the widespread applicability of feminism to modern life. However, I think it has particular purchase on the issue of fetal tissue research, at least in America. While it is a cliché that America is a morally pluralistic country, it is also the case that this pluralism is "dappled" in the sense that there are regions where the balance of different political, religious, and moral beliefs tends to shift in their concentrations.[46] In this moral landscape, one could imagine, for example, that the majority of women in Alabama may come to believe that fetal tissue research is at best dangerous and harmful. Posit further that more women are granted more power in legislative and policy development in government and other institutions. If this were to happen, and further, these powerful women were to act to constrain the choices of other women based on their free exercise of their convictions, how would such a move be inconsistent with basic feminist tenants? And such a scenario need not take place in Alabama, Arkansas, or Alaska.

Consider California: for years the state saw an increase in the number of nonvaccinated children and concomitant infectious outbreaks. In 2015 the state implemented new legislation, Senate Bill No. 277, requiring all public school educated children to be vaccinated without permitting the religious or philosophical exemptions that were previously common. The motivation behind this legislation was its public health benefits, but it straightforwardly curtailed the freedoms of some women and men to make choices for their children, which was justified by the greater good.

Again, if we presume that this type of legislative activity is consistent with the widespread values and preferences held by women, and further that women are in the political positions to champion such restrictions on freedom, then how would such political changes be inconsistent with basic tenants of feminism? In the case of fetal tissue research, the more women experience the choices of whether to donate and discuss them openly together—both activities being entirely consistent with increased adoption of feminist principles—the limited research available suggests that this could lead to constraints on the practices of donating and performing research on fetal tissue.

Perhaps the best response to this line of argument is to return to arguments like those of Schonfeld, Merton, and Ells and colleagues on the nature of "protection." Schonfeld urges readers to be skeptical and thoughtful when interpreting policies designed to protect women and children. Merton and Ells and colleagues' arguments convey that the best way to conceptualize autonomy is in terms of the networks of relationships the bearer of autonomy participates in, which serves to clarify the meaning of autonomous choice in the pragmatic context of that person's existence. In a similar vein, an analytic feminist framework may be interpreted as prioritizing the interests of women *and* other marginalized groups, rather than solely women, who may not, in a possible future, remain marginalized as a group.[47] Perhaps, with this approach in mind, one might respond to this line of argument by calling for continued attention on the effects of policymaking on marginalized persons, regardless of whether most women hold the view that fetal tissue research ought to be significantly constrained. So perhaps radically adopting such positions would be an adequate antidote to the sort of hegemonic use of power by some women over others that I worry about. Perhaps, then, there remains room for optimism about the prospects for a feminist defense of fetal tissue research.

Conclusion

There currently seems to be no end on the horizon for debates about the moral permissibility of embryonic and fetal tissue research, including whether it ought to be supported using public funds. I have advanced the view that appealing to a feminist framework provides compelling arguments against the best available published arguments in support of current U.S. restrictions on fetal tissue research. Analytic feminists emphasize relational autonomy, attending to the biases incorporated into existing policymaking, and prioritizing the interests of women and other marginalized persons when developing and implementing government regulations. I have defended the claim that this framework provides compelling support for fetal tissue research against those who believe otherwise.

However, this support is not without reservations. For one, a feminist framework might conceivably entail that if most women agree there ought to be restrictions on fetal tissue research then this provides warrant for those restrictions. Also, I recognize that analytic feminism is a framework that may be poorly understood by those in a position to affect change in policymaking or that it may be unreasonably dismissed as an ethical framework. However, to concede such moves would be to abandon reason in social and political discourse. Thus, I hope that reason will prevail, and in time social consensus will emerge in support of fetal tissue research, so long as such research is performed with the appropriate, authentic, and informed consent of the women who participate as subjects and who have the authority to elect that the tissues they create be used for research purposes.

Acknowledgments

Thank you to Joseph John, Toby Schonfeld, and Johanna Schoen for their assistance and inspiration in the researching and writing of this paper.

Notes

1. Alta R. Charo, "Fetal Tissue Fallout," *New England Journal of Medicine* 373, no. 10 (2015): 8890–8891, https://doi.org/10.1056/NEJMp1510279, here 8890.
2. Charo, "Fetal Tissue Fallout."
3. Thomas V. Cunningham, "What Justifies the United States Ban on Federal Funding for Nonreproductive Cloning?" *Medicine, Health Care, and Philosophy* 16, no. 4 (2013): 825–841, https://doi.org/10.1007/s11019-013-9465-5.
4. U.S. Department of Health and Human Services, "Statement from the Department of Health and Human Services," June 5, 2019, https://www.hhs.gov/about/news/2019/06/05/statement-from-the-department-of-health-and-human-services.html.
5. Katie Watson, *Scarlet A: The Ethics, Law, and Politics of Ordinary Abortion* (New York: Oxford University Press, 2018).

6. Thomas J. Babbo, "Begging the Question: Fetal Tissue Research, the Protection of Human Subjects, and the Banality of Evil," *DePaul Journal of Health Care Law* 3, no. 3 (2000): 383–410, https://via.library.depaul.edu/jhcl/vol3/iss3/2, here 388.

7. The history of how legal, theological, philosophical, and other forms of reasoning came to bear on public bioethical debates and policymaking is rich and varied. For a full discussion, see David Rothman, *Strangers at the Bedside: A History of How Law and Bioethics Transformed Medical Decision Making* (New York: Basic Books, 1992).

8. Babbo, "Begging the Question," 395 (emphasis added).

9. Babbo, "Begging the Question," 407.

10. 45 C.F.R. § 46.116, 2018.

11. 45 C.F.R. § 46.204, 2018.

12. 45 C.F.R. § 46.206, 2018.

13. Babbo, "Begging the Question," 409 (emphasis added).

14. Cunningham, "What Justifies the United States Ban."

15. Babbo, "Begging the Question," 405. It is worth mentioning that Babbo equivocates the distinguishable concepts in clinical ethics here between *surrogate decision makers*, who make choices for adults who previously had decisional capacity and have lost it, and *parental decision makers*, who make choices for children who have yet to develop sufficiently to make their own choices but who are expected to do so in the future. See Micah D. Hester, "Ethical Issues in Pediatrics," in *Guidance for Healthcare Ethics Committees*, ed. D. M. Hester and T. Schonfield, 114–121 (Cambridge: Cambridge University Press, 2012). Although these distinctions need not be made explicit for the purposes of the current argument, Babbo's claim here also begs questions regarding whether these distinctions should be made, which could have important implications if his approach were to be assumed in the context of medical decision making. Moreover, singling out the mother is not only convenient for his argument but also assumes that others (i.e., the father) have no interest in an abortion. Louis Guenin makes very plain that it is about the progenitors (the men and women who come together in all sorts of biological and social relationships to procreate and parent) who should be the moral authorities regarding how these tissues are used. See Louis Guenin, *The Morality of Embryo Use* (Cambridge: Cambridge University Press, 2008). Finally, women who have abortions do indeed argue that they have the best interest of the fetus in mind. See Johanna Schoen, "Abortion Care as Moral Work," *Journal of Modern European History* 17, no. 3 (2019): 262–279, https://doi.org/10.1177/1611894419854304.

16. Paula Abrams, "The Bad Mother: Stigma, Abortion, and Surrogacy," *Journal of Law, Medicine and Ethics* 43, no. 2 (2015): 179–191, https://doi.org/10.1111/jlme.12231.

17. The history of arguments about the moral status of fetuses and embryos is lengthy and has become caught up in recent decades with questions of the ethics of science and technology. See Jane Maienschein, *Whose View of Life?* (Cambridge, MA: Harvard University Press, 2009). It is outside the scope of this discussion to work through the nuances of these debates; however, readers are directed to Peter Singer, Helga Kuhse, Stephen Buckle, Karen Dawson, and Pascal Kasimba, eds., *Embryo Experimentation: Ethical, Legal, and Social Issues* (New York: Cambridge University Press, 1993) and Suzanne Holland, Karen Lebacqz, and Laurie Zoloth, eds., *The Human Embryonic Stem Cell Debate: Science, Ethics, and Public Policy* (Cambridge, MA: MIT Press, 2001) for anthologies on these issues.

18. Scholarship on the issue of abortion in the United States is substantial. A history of abortion practices and scholarship before and after *Roe v. Wade* can be found in

Johanna Schoen, *Abortion After Roe* (Chapel Hill: University of North Carolina Press, 2015). Many philosophical arguments regarding the moral permissibility of abortion were advanced in the early 1970s, with Judith Jarvis Thomson, "A Defense of Abortion," *Philosophy and Public Affairs* 1, no. 1 (1971): 47–66, https://www.jstor.org /stable/2265091, being the paradigmatic example. Another example is Don Marquis, "Why Abortion is Immoral," *Journal of Philosophy* 86, no. 4 (1989): 183–202, https:// doi.org/10.2307/2026961, which garnered many responses, such as Ann E. Cudd, "Sensationalized Philosophy: A Reply to Marquis's 'Why Abortion is Immoral,'" *Journal of Philosophy* 87, no. 5 (1990): 262–264. His article also contributed to a resurgence in interest in the ethics of abortion (e.g., Rosalind Hursthouse, "Virtue Theory and Abortion," *Philosophy and Public Affairs* 20, no. 3 (1991): 223–246, https:// www.jstor.org/stable/2265432) that continues to the current day. See Raanan Gillon, "Is There a New Ethics of Abortion?" supplement 2, *Journal of Medical Ethics* 27 (2001): ii5–ii9, https://doi.org/10.1136/jme.27.suppl_2.ii5; Elizabeth Harman, "Creation Ethics: The Moral Status of Early Fetuses and the Ethics of Abortion," *Philosophy and Public Affairs* 28, no. 4 (1999): 310–324, https://www.jstor.org/stable /2672875; Francis J. Beckwith, *Defending Life: A Moral and Legal Case Against Abortion Choice* (New York: Cambridge University Press, 2007). Legal scholarship on abortion jurisprudence is rich and wide ranging. For reference, readers are directed to David Masci and Ira C. Lupu, "A History of Key Abortion Rulings of the US Supreme Court," *Pew Research Center*, January 16, 2013, https://www.pewforum.org /2013/01/16/a-history-of-key-abortion-rulings-of-the-us-supreme-court/, and the following exemplars on the topic as well as citations therein: John A. Robertson, "Gestational Burdens and Fetal Status: Justifying *Roe v. Wade*," *American Journal of Law and Medicine* 13, no. 2–3 (1987): 189–212, https://doi.org/10.1017/S0098858800008339; Reva Siegal, "Reasoning from the Body: A Historical Perspective on Abortion Regulation and Questions of Equal Protection," *Stanford Law Review* 44 (1992): 261–381, https://law.yale.edu/sites/default/files/documents/pdf/Faculty/Siegel_Reasoning FromTheBody.pdf; Wendy K. Mariner, "The Supreme Court, Abortion, and the Jurisprudence of Class," *American Journal of Public Health* 82, no. 11 (1992): 1556–1562, https://doi.org/10.2105/ajph.82.11.1556; Pamela Laufer-Ukeles, "Reproductive Choices and Informed Consent Fetal Interests, Women's Identity, and Relational Autonomy," *American Journal of Law and Medicine* 37, no. 4 (2011): 567–623, https://doi.org/10 .1177/009885881103700403.

19. My approach is consistent with Suzanne Holland's which grounds a conceptual analysis of the morality of fetal tissue research in a framework of analytic feminism. However, Holland focuses on stem cells, which may be derived from fetal tissues as well as other sources rather than tissues derived from human fetuses. Holland also is concerned with Clinton era policies restricting the use of stem cells and similar biotechnologies that do not concern us in this discussion. Finally, Holland's analysis emphasizes the possible implications of stem cell research to women and marginalized persons, which I suppress in this discussion but is worthy of significant consideration. See Suzanne Holland, "Beyond the Embryo: A Feminist Appraisal of the Embryonic Stem Cell Debate," in Holland et al., eds., 73–86, *Human Embryonic Stem Cell Debate*.

20. Jennifer Nedelsky, "Reconceiving Autonomy: Sources, Thoughts and Possibilities," *Yale Journal of Law and Feminism* 1, no. 7 (1989): 7–36, https://digitalcommons.law .yale.edu/yjlf/vol1/iss1/5.

21. Carolyn Ells, Matthew R. Hunt, and Jane Chambers-Evans, "Relational Autonomy as an Essential Component of Patient-Centered Care," *International Journal of*

Feminist Approaches to Bioethics 4, no. 2 (2011): 79–101, https://doi.org/10.2979 /intjfemappbio.4.2.79, here 86.

22. Pamela Laufer-Ukeles also makes a similar point in legal scholarship concerning reproductive decision making (see Laufer-Ukeles, "Reproductive Choices and Informed Consent").

23. Note that this argumentative strategy may be deployed to an opposing conclusion: Guenin persuasively argues that donations of cellular material, such as embryonic or fetal material, should be treated like other donations for scientific research in the sense that it is on the authority of the individuals who biologically produce that material that the donation is morally justified. Guenin looks back to the progenitors of these cells and tissues—namely, the men and women who produce them via copulation or in vitro fertilization—and argues that they have the unique authority to choose whether and how those cells may be used for the purposes of research. In this regard, Guenin's approach fits nicely with the findings reported by Parry discussed later. See Sarah Parry, "(Re-)constructing Embryos in Stem Cell Research: Exploring the Meaning of Embryos for People Involved in Fertility Treatments," *Social Science and Medicine* 62 (2006): 2349–2359, https://doi.org/10.1016/j.socscimed.2005.10.024.

24. Ells et al., "Relational Autonomy"; Tom L. Beauchamp and James F. Childress, *Principles of Bioethics*, 5th ed. (New York: Oxford University Press, 2001).

25. Vanessa Merton, "The Exclusion of Pregnant, Pregnable, and Once-Pregnable People (a.k.a. Women) from Biomedical Research," *American Journal of Law and Medicine* 19, no. 4 (1993): 369–451, https://doi.org/10.1017/S0098858800010121.

26. Merton, "Exclusion of Pregnant," 360.

27. Rebecca Dresser, "Wanted: Single, White Male for Medical Research," *Hastings Center Report* 22, no. 1 (1993): 24–29, https://doi.org/10.2307/3562720; Nancy Kass, Holly A. Taylor, and Patricia A. King, "Harms of Excluding Pregnant Women from Clinical Research: The Case of HIV Infected Pregnant Women," *Journal of Law, Medicine and Ethics* 24, no. 1 (1996): 36–46, https://doi.org/10.1111/j.1748-720X.1996 .tb01831.x; Anne Drapkin Lyerly, Margaret Olivia Little, and Ruth Faden, "The Second Wave: Toward Responsible Inclusion of Pregnant Women in Research," *IJFAB: International Journal of Feminist Approaches to Bioethics* 1, no. 2 (2008): 5–22, https://doi.org/10.3138/ijfab.1.2.5.

28. Lyerly et al., "Second Wave," 5.

29. Toby Schonfeld, "The Perils of Protection: Vulnerability and Women in Clinical Research," *Theoretical Medicine and Bioethics* 34, no. 3 (2013): 189–206, https://doi .org/10.1007/s11017-013-9258-0, 189.

30. Schonfeld, "The Perils of Protection," 194.

31. Schonfeld, "The Perils of Protection," 195.

32. Schonfeld, "The Perils of Protection," 200.

33. One may be excused for wondering whether reflecting on how women, health care providers, and researchers choose to dispose of fetal tissue is a merely academic exercise. It is not, as recent, unconstitutional, and failed attempts by the Texas legislature to compel women to bury fetal tissues resulting from miscarriages or abortions show. See Joanna Grossman, "Texas Judges Give Unconstitutional Fetal Remains Law a Proper Burial," *Verdict*, September 11, 2018, https://verdict.justia.com/2018/09/11 /texas-judges-give-unconstitutional-fetal-remains-law-a-proper-burial.

34. Natalie Stoljar, "Feminist Perspectives on Autonomy," *Stanford Encyclopedia of Philosophy*, ed. Edward N. Zalta (Fall 2015 edition), https://plato.stanford.edu/archives /fall2015/entries/feminism-autonomy/.

35. Ann Garry, "Analytic Feminism," *Stanford Encyclopedia of Philosophy*, ed. Edward N. Zalta (Fall 2018 edition), https://plato.stanford.edu/archives/fall2018/entries/femap proach-analytic/.

36. Julie Kent, "The Fetal Tissue Economy: From the Abortion Clinic to the Stem Cell Laboratory," *Social Science and Medicine* 67 (2008): 1747–1756, https://doi.org/10.1016/j.socscimed.2008.09.027.

37. Fionn Anderson, Anna Glasier, Jonathan Ross, and David T. Baird, "Attitudes of Women to Fetal Tissue Research," *Journal of Medical Ethics* 20 (1994): 36–40, https://doi.org/10.1136/jme.20.1.36; Naomi Pfeffer, "What British Women Say Matters to Them About Donating an Aborted Fetus to Stem Cell Research: A Focus Group Study," *Social Science and Medicine* (2008): 2544–2554, https://doi.org/10.1016/j.socscimed.2008.01.050; Parry, "(Re-)constructing Embryos"; Clare Williams, "Framing the Fetus in Medical Work: Rituals and Practices," *Social Science and Medicine* 60 (2005): 2085–2095, https://doi.org/10.1016/j.socscimed.2004.09.003.

38. Anderson et al., "Attitudes of Women," 36.

39. Pfeffer, "What British Women Say," 2548.

40. Pfeffer, "What British Women Say," 2551.

41. Pfeffer, "What British Women Say," 2550–2551.

42. Pfeffer, "What British Women Say," 2553.

43. Anderson et al., "Attitudes of Women."

44. Parry, "(Re-)constructing Embryos," 2354.

45. Parry, "(Re-)constructing Embryos."

46. Nancy Cartwright develops the concept of a "dappled world" to describe the way lawlike regularities hold in the world. My usage of "dappled" is intended to echo hers, in that it conveys that the moral landscape of American society is not merely pluralistic, where many different views are plausible and believed to different degrees. Rather, the moral landscape is dappled, in that certain locales are quite cosmopolitan while in other locales the range of socially acceptable views is far more constrained. See Nancy Cartwright, *The Dappled World: A Study of the Boundaries of Science* (New York: Cambridge University Press, 1999); and William E. Connolly, *Pluralism* (Durhan, NC: Duke University Press, 2005).

47. Holland, "Beyond the Embryo."

Chapter 12

Definitions of Viability and Their Meaning for Neonatal Care

John Colin Partridge

In my daily life as a neonatologist working in the neonatal intensive care unit (NICU), I deal more often with the presumption of life and potential viability than with presumed nonviability. I work in a world where perinatal counseling and decision making must transition from an antenatal (before birth) focus on the fetus and mother to a postnatal (after birth) focus predominantly on the neonate (the newborn). Given the overall success of obstetric and neonatal intensive care, decision making about life-support in the NICU focuses far more often on the quality of life the surviving infant will have than on viability—whether the infant can survive. In my world, birth and neonatal decisions hinge predominantly on the anticipated future status of a specific fetus—whose outcome I can rarely predict accurately—and on the balance of maternal and fetal rights. After birth, rights of the newborn are arguably less controversial. But they still come into question for infants whose potential depends completely on the technology available and the decisions that we make for them.

Neonates are not autonomous. They lack the capacity to consider the options and to make decisions about medical care for themselves. We turn to proxies, typically parents and the medical team, to make decisions for the neonate. In addition, courts, legislative bodies, ethics committees, religious leaders, and potential interest groups may be brought into decisions made on behalf of the neonate regarding resuscitation and life-sustaining therapies. With the help of a variety of medical technologies—from steroids to resuscitation to kinder and gentler types of mechanical ventilation that help prevent chronic lung disease—we are today able to keep babies alive who would have died in the past.

Today we are able to employ a broad array of life-saving interventions for premature infants. Indeed, we can do so much that "miracle babies" have been created. In 2006, Amillia Taylor was born at twenty-one and 6/7 weeks and 280 grams. Amillia was on websites at least through 2008, her second birthday, raising questions about treatment guidelines, parental choices, and the political context surrounding discussions of viability. "Guidelines continue to be controversial," Marilee Allen and Betty Vohr noted, "and the families of infants born at 21 or 22 weeks of gestational age may pressure clinicians to resuscitate these infants. This situation is becoming more common as a result of the increasing rate of premature births, advanced maternal age, the increased use of assisted reproductive technology, and the publicity about 'miracle babies' in the media."[1] However, in our institution and in most others nationwide, gestational ages of twenty-one and twenty-two weeks are considered nonviable.

An obstetrician cannot definitively predict if a fetus or embryo is going to be normal or abnormal. A significant number of fetuses die before they see the light of day. And in my universe, half of the most immature preterm neonates we take care of in the neonatal intensive care unit do not survive to hospital discharge. They fail to survive despite every technologic measure we can, and do, offer. But, in my opinion, what drives decision making as neonatologists, parents, and potentially society is the cohort of neonates who survive, but do so significantly damaged.

In approaching decisions about the appropriateness of neonatal intensive care, the first question we ask is one of physiology: can the infant survive? Here, there are objective criteria for infants who cannot survive a lethal diagnosis in which all interventions will fail to ameliorate the condition and save the infant's life. Examples would be extreme immaturity, lethal anomalies, brain death, and anencephaly. In perinatal counseling for infants with severe conditions that are not lethal, we deal with quantitative viability derived from survival statistics reported in the medical literature for similar infants. Outcomes are reported as group outcomes because the range of potential viability for a specific infant is difficult to estimate. We are talking about what is biologically possible—what the most probable outcomes are. We ask, What are the chances? When is intervention futile? These questions require subjective assessment. What is the percent success rate for a medical intervention in intensive care?

I liken this to being on an airplane. No one is going to get on an airplane that has a 20 percent chance of landing safely. But women and their fetuses are already on that plane. Compared with certain death, they are looking at a 20 percent chance of survival as a favorable outcome. We are also talking about group-specific outcomes, the presence or absence of specific risk factors, and added speculation as to the specific outcome for that infant. When I am talking about statistics to a potential mother, I am, in fact, not talking about her baby. I cannot predict *her* infant's outcome with any precision. Rather, I am talking about the statistical outcome of a hundred babies. Worse, long-term outcome data stem from data derived up to a decade before, and our assessments, practices, and outcomes change over time.

Even more controversial is the question of qualitative futility. Who should we or should we not treat based on the expected quality of life? This is judgment based. We look at burdens of treatment and an infant's presumed quality of life. For example, is the quality of life unacceptable with a severe chromosomal disorder or with catastrophic brain injury from birth asphyxia? How far should we be willing to go to ensure that the infant survives when all prognostic indicators point to a life with profound disabilities? At what point can a choice for withdrawal of support go too far down the slippery slope? Outcomes have certainly improved significantly for perinatal asphyxia and even more markedly for extremely premature infants. For infants at extreme immature gestation, twenty-two to twenty-five weeks, outcomes have improved overall between 1995 and 2020.[2] But while we are now able to do much more at twenty-five weeks' gestation, there is much less improvement in infants below twenty-four weeks' gestation. The American College of Obstetricians and Gynecologists and the American Academy of Pediatrics (AAP) recommend "routine" perinatal intensive management of infants at twenty-three weeks' gestation.[3] However, we strongly recommend against resuscitation and NICU care, as well as limiting resuscitation and intensive care based on criteria that maximize survival and minimize morbidity. If both parents wish to go against our recommendation at twenty-three weeks, however, we allow parents to opt for more intensive care.

Still, for the past three decades this has been our concern: Are we saving a larger proportion of infants who are damaged and forced to lead a life—because we have chosen life for them—during which they will face significant disability that will impair both their own and their families' potential? About one-third to as many as half of the most premature babies have severe disabilities: severe blindness, hearing impairment requiring amplification, an inability to walk without support, cerebral palsy, or significant cognitive neurological deficits. Is it in the best interest of the fetus to survive with such disabilities? If we analyze the self-reported health frequencies of adolescent and young adult survivors of extreme prematurity, their reports of being affected by health-related life attributes (sensory, mobility, emotion, cognition, self-care, pain) show very little statistical differences compared with the quality of life in adolescents who were not born prematurely.[4] This is a strong indication that the life as lived is not as bad as we think. In addition, there are also data demonstrating that neonatologists and obstetricians hold more pessimistic perspectives on survival and quality of life than the parents and survivors themselves.[5]

Clearly beneficial treatment begins somewhere at or after twenty-three weeks, and the benefit increases with increased gestation.[6] At the same time, the concept of futility diminishes at twenty-three weeks.[7] If we look at resuscitation preferences, very few people expect or select resuscitation at twenty-two weeks. Beginning at twenty-six weeks, most parents and physicians prefer or expect full resuscitation. The shift occurs around twenty-four to twenty-five weeks where we see a significant split between parents desiring resuscitation and physicians preferring no resuscitation. Similarly, as it relates to decisions between limited versus comfort care, before twenty-six weeks' gestation the parents prefer more aggressive care than physicians or nurses.

As late as the early 1970s, infants with trisomy 21 and correctable anomalies were often denied nutrition or surgical correction based on the "financial and emotional burden on the rest of the family." In 1971, after a study of 524 infants with meningomyelocele, J. Lorber proposed the first written criteria for selective nonintervention, specifically for infants with high-level spina bifida.[8] In their landmark 1973 article, Raymond Duff and A.G.M. Campbell reported that 54 percent of deaths in a special care nursery followed nonintervention decisions by parents and physicians. Thus, parents and physicians were willing to opt for nonintervention when the prognosis was hopeless or the future potential for "meaningful life" extremely poor.[9] Again, in 1994 Steve Wall and I reported that in our nursery 74 percent of NICU deaths followed decisions to limit treatment for severely compromised infants.[10]

But decisions to limit treatment for severely compromised infants have also become political and led to congressional intervention. In 1984, Congress passed the so-called Baby Doe Regulations. The law mandated that states receiving federal money for child abuse programs develop procedures to report medical neglect, which the law defines as the withholding of treatment—regardless of the wishes of the parents—unless a baby is irreversibly comatose or the treatment for the newborn's survival is "virtually futile." In 2002, Congress passed the Born Alive Infant Protection Act (BAIPA), which extends legal protection to all infants born alive—indeed, intended for cases where infants were born alive after a failed abortion—regardless of gestational age. The law was posited as a political action to define the constitutional rights of any infant born with any sign of life, regardless of the intent of the pregnancy or the method of delivery. I am not sure what, if anything, can—let alone should—be done with a live born eighteen- or twenty-one-weeker. In a survey of California neonatologists, only 7 percent believed that this law should be enforced.[11] Sixty-five percent of California neonatologists thought the law would affect options to withhold or withdraw life support. Eighty-nine percent believed that it would prohibit palliative care *only* options.

The federal act requires a screening examination and appropriate medical care. However, screening examinations are not routinely performed below twenty-two weeks' gestation, and any examination at that gestation provides absolutely no prognostic information on survival, let alone on quality of life. Some people have argued that we should see what happens when we offer a "trial of therapy." This might push physicians to resuscitate extremely premature infants and admit them to the NICU for a trial of therapy while the prognosis for survival and for anticipated long-term morbidity is being refined. This would increase NICU admissions, diagnostic tests, and overall costs of care. Analysis following passage of the BAIPA did show a small but statistically significant change in the fetal and live-birth death rates for infants considered previable but only among the most immature at 17 weeks' gestation.

The BAIPA regulation called for "appropriate medical care," without specifying what is appropriate for infants at differing gestational ages (let alone for other conditions where viability comes into question). Certainly, it is our charge to do everything appropriate to maximize survival. The AAP Neonatal Resuscitation Program guidelines suggest it may be inappropriate to resuscitate infants younger than twenty-three weeks, with a birth weight lower than 400 grams, or with anencephaly or confirmed trisomy 13 or 18. At the time of delivery, the guidelines note, "decisions about withholding or discontinuing treatment that is considered futile may be considered by the medical care providers in conjunction with the parents acting in the best interests of their child."[12]

If we look at data from a survey of informed neonatologists, we find survival estimates of 25 to 30 percent for a preterm infant born at twenty-two weeks or an infant with hypoxic ischemic encephalopathy (HIE)—newborn brain damage caused by oxygen deprivation and limited blood flow—or trisomy 13, conditions that the AAP suggests are severe enough to consider nonintervention an appropriate choice. If this survival estimate is taken as a quantitative limit of viability, it seems stunningly high. On the other end of the spectrum, anencephaly was perceived by these neonatologists as nonviable.

And finally, when would physicians be willing to override parental decision making? In our survey, at twenty-two weeks' gestation, 50 percent of physicians reported they would be willing to override parents wishing for NICU care. On the other side at twenty-four weeks' gestation, 41 percent of physicians reported they would be willing to override parents' preference for comfort care.

After looking at overall infant outcomes in a theoretical model of all U.S. deliveries in the year 2009, we found the following: if you resuscitate everyone, more infants survive, but a significant number have significant neurological compromises. If you don't resuscitate, almost everybody dies. At twenty-three to 23 6/7th weeks' gestation, it costs $1.2 billion to resuscitate every infant, and it was not beneficial to women. It lowered women's quality of life due to the significant financial and emotional burdens of caregiving, leading to depression, stress, loss of employment, and marital problems. But for utility analysts, any neonatal-based assessment is mathematically positive. Infants survive perfectly at a utility of 1 or die with a utility of 0. Thus, there is no life worse than death. And using a widely accepted definition of <$100,000 per quality-adjusted life-year, if you combine these two data points, aggressive neonatal care for twenty-three-week infants becomes "cost-effective," despite disabilities among some survivors. For utility analysts, the benefits from improved neonatal survival outweigh the negative effects on the mother.[13]

In sum, there are three categories: infants that most of us agree should be resuscitated and receive intensive care, those that should not, and then a grey zone at twenty-three to twenty-four weeks and at 500 to 650 grams where disagreement about appropriateness of intensive care is both ethical and legitimate. There really is no consensus. We have more data, if not answers, on the "appropriateness" of some interventions. Neither government policy nor case law clarifies the matter. Practices are varied, inconsistent, and often paternalistic. It matters where and into whose care you are born. Quality of life, more often than physiologic viability, drives decisions about life-support in the NICU.

Notes

1. Betty R. Vohr and Marilee Allen, "Extreme Prematurity—The Continuing Dilemma," *New England Journal of Medicine* 352, no. 1 (2005): 71–72, https://doi.org/10.1056/nejme048323, here 71.

2. Noelle Younge, Ricki F. Goldstein, Carla M. Bann, et al., "Survival and Neurodevelopmental Outcomes among Periviable Infants," *New England Journal of Medicine*, 376, no. 7 (2017): 617–628, https://doi.org/10.1056/nejmoa1605566.

3. T.N.K. Raju, B. M. Mercer, D. J. Burchfield, and G. F. Joseph, "Periviable Birth: Executive Summary of a Joint Workshop by the *Eunice Kennedy Shriver* National Institute of Child Health and Human Development, Society for Maternal-Fetal Medicine, American Academy of Pediatrics, and American College of Obstetricians and Gynecologists," *Journal of Perinatology* 34, no. 5 (2014): 333–342, https://doi.org/10.1038/jp.2014.70.

4. Saroj Saigal, David Feeny, Peter Rosenbaum, William Furlong, Elizabeth Burrows, and Barbara Stoskopf, "Self-perceived Health Status and Health-Related Quality of Life of Extremely Low-Birth-Weight Infants at Adolescence," *JAMA* 276, no. 6 (1996): 453–459, 10.1001/jama.1996.03540060029031.

5. David L. Streiner, Saroj Saigal, Elizabeth Burrows, Barbara Stoskopf, and Peter Rosenbaum, "Attitudes of Parents and Health Care Professionals Toward Active Treatment of Extremely Premature Infants," *Pediatrics* 108, no. 1 (2001): 152–157, https://doi.org/10.1542/peds.108.1.152; Steven B. Morse, James L. Haywood, Robert L. Goldenberg, Janet Bronstein, Kathleeen G. Nelson, and Waldemar A. Carlo, "Estimation of Neonatal Outcome and Perinatal Therapy Use," *Pediatrics* 105, no. 5 (2000):1046–1050, https://doi.org/10.1542/peds.105.5.1046.

6. Jane E. Brumbaugh, Nellie I. Hansen, Edward F. Bell, et al., "Outcomes of Extremely Preterm Infants with Birth Weight Less Than 400 g," *JAMA Pediatrics* 173, no. 5 (2019): 434–445, https://doi.org/10.1001/jamapediatrics.2019.0180.

7. Jaideep Singh, Jon Fanaroff, Bree Andrews, Leslie Caldarelli, Joanne Lagatta, Susan Plesha-Troyke, John Lantos, and William Meadow, "Resuscitation in the 'Gray Zone' of Viability: Determining Physician Preferences and Predicting Infant Outcomes," *Pediatrics* 120, no. 3 (2007): 519–526, https://doi.org/10.1542/peds.2006-2966.

8. J. Lorber, "Results of Treatment of Myelomeningocele: An Analysis of 524 Unselected Cases, with Special Reference to Possible Selection for Treatment," *Developmental Medicine and Child Neurology* 13, no. 3 (1971): 279–303, https://doi.org/10.1111/j.1469-8749.1971.tb03264.x.

9. Raymond S. Duff and A.G.M. Campbell, "Moral and Ethical Dilemmas in the Special Care Nursery," *New England Journal of Medicine* 289, no. 17 (1973): 890–894, https://doi.org/10.1056/nejm197310252891705.

10. Stephen N. Wall and John Colin Partridge, "Death in the Intensive Care Nursery: Physician Practice of Withdrawing and Withholding Life Support," *Pediatrics* 99, no. 1 (1997): 64–70, https://doi.org/10.1542/peds.99.1.64.

11. J. Colin Partridge, Mya D. Sendowski, Eleanor A. Drey, and Alma M. Martinez, "Resuscitation of Likely Nonviable Newborns: Would Neonatology Practices in California Change if the Born-Alive Infants Protection Act Were Enforced?" *Pediatrics* 123, no. 4 (2009): 1088–1094, https://doi.org/10.1542/peds.2008-0643.

12. American Academy of Pediatrics Committee on Fetus and Newborn and Edward F. Bell, "Noninitiation or Withdrawal of Intensive Care for High-Risk Newborns," *Pediatrics* 119, no. 2 (2007): 401–403, https://doi.org/10.1542/peds.2006-3180; see also Gary M. Weiner and Jeanette Zaichkin, eds., *Textbook of Neonatal Resuscitation*, 7th ed. (Elk Grove Village, IL: American Academy of Pediatrics, 2016). The AAP NRP 2011 guidelines noted, "If the responsible physicians believe that there is no chance for survival, initiation of resuscitation is not an ethical treatment option and should not be offered. Examples include birth at a confirmed gestational age of less than twenty-two weeks' gestation and some congenital malformations and chromosomal anomalies. In conditions associated with a high risk of mortality or significant burden of morbidity for the baby, caregivers should discuss the risks and benefits of life-sustaining treatment and allow the parents to participate in the decision whether attempting resuscitation is in their baby's best interest. If there is agreement between the parents and the caregivers that intensive medical care will not improve the chances for the newborn's survival or will pose an unacceptable burden on the child, it is ethical to provide compassionate palliative care and not initiate resuscitation." Jeanette Zaichkin and Gary M, Weiner, "Neonatal Resuscitation Program (NRP) 2011: New Science, New Strategies," *Advances in Neonatal Care* 11, no. 1 (Feb. 2011): 43–51, https://doi.org/10.1097/ANC.0b013e31820e429f.

13. Peter J. Neumann and Joshua T. Cohen, "QALYs in 2018—Advantages and Concerns," *JAMA* 319, no. 24 (2018): 2473–2474, https://doi.org/10.1001/jama.2018.6072.

Notes on Contributors

Terry Beresford, 1929–2014, trained abortion counselors and held a variety of positions in family planning and counseling, including director of the Preterm Center for Reproductive Health in Washington, DC, and director of counseling at Planned Parenthood of Maryland.

Curtis Boyd, MD, is the founder of Southwestern Women's Options, which offers abortion care in Texas and New Mexico.

Renee Chelian is the founder and Executive Director at Northland Family Planning Centers with three clinics providing abortion care in the Detroit area.

Thomas V. Cunningham is the medical bioethics director at Kaiser Permanente in Los Angeles, California.

Michelle Debbink, MD, PhD, is a maternal fetal medicine specialist at the University of Utah.

Sara Dubow is a professor of history at Williams College and the author of *Ourselves Unborn: Fetal Meanings in Modern America*.

Glenna Halvorson-Boyd has a PhD in human and organizational development and works as a counselor, trainer, and consultant in the field of abortion care.

Lisa H. Harris is a professor in the Department of Obstetrics and Gynecology at the University of Michigan with a secondary appointment in the Department of Women's Studies.

Jane A. Hassinger, LCSW, DCSW, is an emeritus professor at the University of Michigan, Ann Arbor, Institute for Research on Women and Gender.

Marc Heller is a retired, board-certified obstetrician and gynecologist who provided abortion care for Planned Parenthood in upstate New York.

Lisa A. Martin, PhD, is an associate professor of Health Policy Studies and director of Women's and Gender Studies at the University of Michigan at Dearborn.

Amy Hagstrom Miller is the founder, president, and CEO of Whole Woman's Health, which operates eight clinics providing abortion care across the country.

John Colin Partridge is a retired professor of pediatrics and neonatologist at the University of California at San Francisco.

Johanna Schoen is professor of history at Rutgers University at New Brunswick and the author of *Abortion after Roe*.

Shelley Sella is a retired board-certified obstetrician and gynecologist who provided abortion care at Southwestern Women's Options.

Morris Turner, 1948–2014, was an obstetrician and gynecologist at the University of Pittsburgh Medical Center in Pittsburgh, Pennsylvania, where he provided abortion care.

Shannon K. Withycombe is an associate professor of history at the University of New Mexico and the author of *Lost: Miscarriage in Nineteenth Century America* (Rutgers University Press, 2018).

Index

Abbott, Greg, 61

Aborted Women: Silent No More (Reardon), 73

abortion: as act of compassion, 91–92; as act of conscience, 99–104; antiabortion movement and legalization of, 4; bans on abortion after 20 weeks' gestation, 56; Black genocide and, 24–25; decision to end pregnancy as moral decision, 75–76; as essential health care, 61–62; hyperregulation of affecting connection and community, 58; legalization of, 1–2, 4 (see also *Roe v. Wade*); moral agency of women and, 75–76, 99, 101–104; need to speak about complexities of, 62–64; number of after legalization of, 2; number of before legalization of, 1; state restrictions on, 8–9 (*see also* targeted regulation of abortion providers (TRAP) laws); women's reason for seeking, 76–79. *See also* illegal abortion

Abortion Act of 1967 (Great Britain), 160–162

abortion care: improving, 65–69; meaning of viability in, 105–109

abortion clinics, 49–54; closing of, 63; demand for services and growth of, 3–4; direct action tactics of antiabortion protesters and, 5–6, 17–18; feminists and freestanding, 49, 50; freestanding model, 3, 64; improving abortion care and, 65–69; informed consent instead of counseling at, 47; networks of, 2, 3, 51–52; security for, 29–30; seeking help from police regarding protesters, 17–18; vulnerability to antiabortion laws and regulations, 52–53

abortion committees, hospital, 13, 22

abortion counseling, 67; establishing, 39–48; individual counseling protocol, 100–101; model for, 41–42; at Planned Parenthood, 43–44; at Preterm, 39, 40–43;

as short-term crisis intervention counseling, 42

abortion counselors, hiring, 43–44

abortion narratives, 110–111; ultrasound and, 72–73; women characterized as passive victims or as in need of protection in, 73–74. *See also* fetal narratives

abortion providers, 13–19; difficulties of doing abortion work for, 110–112; effect of hyperregulation on, 56–60; emotional impact of dilation and evacuation procedures on, 75; essay on experience of being, 32–38; experience of sharing silenced stories, 122; fulfilling antiabortion stereotypes, 115–116; harassment of, 6; judging patients, 113; lack of connection to movement advocacy, 121–122; laws requiring admitting privileges to local hospitals for, 56, 60–61; life and death encounters with fetuses and, 116–119; memoirs of becoming and practicing as, 21–31, 99–104; moral uncertainty and, 113–114; murders of, 7–8, 18, 25, 27, 31, 31n4, 105; obligation to pregnant women and respect for fetus, 79; portrayal of by antiabortion movement, 5; reason for providing abortion services, 13, 66; religion and religious intolerance in pro-choice communities and, 114–115; safety concerns for selves and families, 27–29; self-censorship and, 119–120, 128–129; self-silencing of, 111–112; social disapproval experienced by, 17, 32; stories not shared, 111, 113–119; study of feelings and attitudes of, 112–128; tasks of, 38; tension between work experience and pro-choice advocacy, 119–122; violence against, 7–8, 18, 25, 27, 31, 31n4, 101, 105

abortion reform in 1960s, 14

abortion rights movement. *See* pro-choice movement

Available titles in the Critical Issues in Health and Medicine series:

Mark A. Hall and Sara Rosenbaum, eds., *The Health Care "Safety Net" in a Post-Reform World*

Laura L. Heinemann, *Transplanting Care: Shifting Commitments in Health and Care in the United States*

Rebecca J. Hester, *Embodied Politics: Indigenous Migrant Activism, Cultural Competency, and Health Promotion in California*

Laura D. Hirshbein, *American Melancholy: Constructions of Depression in the Twentieth Century*

Laura D. Hirshbein, *Smoking Privileges: Psychiatry, the Mentally Ill, and the Tobacco Industry in America*

Timothy Hoff, *Practice under Pressure: Primary Care Physicians and Their Medicine in the Twenty-first Century*

Beatrix Hoffman, Nancy Tomes, Rachel N. Grob, and Mark Schlesinger, eds., *Patients as Policy Actors*

Ruth Horowitz, *Deciding the Public Interest: Medical Licensing and Discipline*

Powel Kazanjian, *Frederick Novy and the Development of Bacteriology in American Medicine*

Claas Kirchhelle, *Pyrrhic Progress: The History of Antibiotics in Anglo-American Food Production*

Rebecca M. Kluchin, *Fit to Be Tied: Sterilization and Reproductive Rights in America, 1950–1980*

Jennifer Lisa Koslow, *Cultivating Health: Los Angeles Women and Public Health Reform*

Jennifer Lisa Koslow, *Exhibiting Health: Public Health Displays in the Progressive Era*

Susan C. Lawrence, *Privacy and the Past: Research, Law, Archives, Ethics*

Bonnie Lefkowitz, *Community Health Centers: A Movement and the People Who Made It Happen*

Ellen Leopold, *Under the Radar: Cancer and the Cold War*

Barbara L. Ley, *From Pink to Green: Disease Prevention and the Environmental Breast Cancer Movement*

Sonja Mackenzie, *Structural Intimacies: Sexual Stories in the Black AIDS Epidemic*

Stephen E. Mawdsley, *Selling Science: Polio and the Promise of Gamma Globulin*

Frank M. McClellan, *Healthcare and Human Dignity: Law Matters*

Michelle McClellan, *Lady Lushes: Gender, Alcohol, and Medicine in Modern America*

David Mechanic, *The Truth about Health Care: Why Reform Is Not Working in America*

Richard A. Meckel, *Classrooms and Clinics: Urban Schools and the Protection and Promotion of Child Health, 1870–1930*

Terry Mizrahi, *From Residency to Retirement: Physicians' Careers over a Professional Lifetime*

Manon Parry, *Broadcasting Birth Control: Mass Media and Family Planning*

Alyssa Picard, *Making the American Mouth: Dentists and Public Health in the Twentieth Century*

Heather Munro Prescott, *The Morning After: A History of Emergency Contraception in the United States*

Sarah B. Rodriguez, *The Love Surgeon: A Story of Trust, Harm, and the Limits of Medical Regulation*

David J. Rothman and David Blumenthal, eds., *Medical Professionalism in the New Information Age*

Andrew R. Ruis, *Eating to Learn, Learning to Eat: School Lunches and Nutrition Policy in the United States*

James A. Schafer Jr., *The Business of Private Medical Practice: Doctors, Specialization, and Urban Change in Philadelphia, 1900–1940*